AF717282

Healthcare Systems

Series Editor
Jean-Charles Pomerol

Healthcare Systems

Challenges and Opportunities

Edited by

Sondès Chaabane
Etienne Cousein
Philippe Wieser

ISTE

WILEY

First published 2022 in Great Britain and the United States by ISTE Ltd and John Wiley & Sons, Inc.

Apart from any fair dealing for the purposes of research or private study, or criticism or review, as permitted under the Copyright, Designs and Patents Act 1988, this publication may only be reproduced, stored or transmitted, in any form or by any means, with the prior permission in writing of the publishers, or in the case of reprographic reproduction in accordance with the terms and licenses issued by the CLA. Enquiries concerning reproduction outside these terms should be sent to the publishers at the undermentioned address:

ISTE Ltd
27-37 St George's Road
London SW19 4EU
UK

www.iste.co.uk

John Wiley & Sons, Inc.
111 River Street
Hoboken, NJ 07030
USA

www.wiley.com

© ISTE Ltd 2022
The rights of Sondès Chaabane, Etienne Cousein and Philippe Wieser to be identified as the authors of this work have been asserted by them in accordance with the Copyright, Designs and Patents Act 1988.

Any opinions, findings, and conclusions or recommendations expressed in this material are those of the author(s), contributor(s) or editor(s) and do not necessarily reflect the views of ISTE Group.

Library of Congress Control Number: 2021951467

British Library Cataloguing-in-Publication Data
A CIP record for this book is available from the British Library
ISBN 978-1-78630-799-6

MIX
Paper from
responsible sources
FSC® C013604

Contents

Foreword

The first GISEH conference was in 2003 at Hôpital de la Croix-Rousse in Lyon, the result of a collaboration between the PRISMa laboratory at the *Institut National des Sciences Appliquées de Lyon* and the *Pôle Nord des Hospices Civils de Lyon* on the organization and management of operating theatres, which sought to question the adaptability of industrial engineering tools in a hospital setting. At that time, changes to funding of hospital activities through Activity-Based Costing (as part of the *Hôpital 2007* plan) forced healthcare players to refocus on medico-technical platforms that created added value. This first conference attracted 106 participants from France, Belgium, Luxembourg, Switzerland, among others, with around 66 presentations directly addressing issues in the hospital world and in collaboration with hospital workers. GISEH takes is designed to span the fields of engineering, the social sciences and medicine and thus assumes a cross-cutting form.

A little over a year later in 2004, the city of Mons in Belgium hosted the second GISEH at the *Facultés Universitaires Catholique de Mons* (FUCaM). Belgian hospital workers are subject to the same constraints and share the same objectives as their French counterparts, and it is with this in mind that their projects and initial feedback is presented. This second conference was equally successful with about 100 participants and 57 publications. Mons gives its French-speaking dimension to GISEH and thus a greater dynamism.

2006 saw the third GISEH, this time hosted in Luxembourg at the *Centre de Recherche Public Henri Tudor*, which works on health and social security issues in collaboration with numerous hospitals. A total of 190 participants came to listen to 75 presentations. Special issues of the best works were published in French-language journals such as *Logistique et Management*, *La Valeur* or *Gestion Hospitalière*. This third conference cemented GISEH as a significant contributor in discussions on hospitals and healthcare.

The *Ecole Polytechnique de Lausanne* organized the 4th GISEH in 2008. A total of 160 participants, a third of whom were hospital-based, came to listen to 89 presentations. Logistical, operational, informational and decision-making activities were widely discussed and brought together in the GISEH melting pot. The fields under investigation at GISEH conferences were broadening and giving new meaning to the cross-cutting spirit between the engineering, social and medical sciences.

The 5th GISEH was organized in September 2010 at the *Centre Hospitalier Universitaire de Clermont-Ferrand* by LIMOS (*Laboratoire d'Informatique, de Modélisation et d'Optimisation des Systèmes*). Two hundred participants, including 73 hospital staff, considered new structures in order to meet the objectives set for them, in terms of patient satisfaction, quality of care, cost reduction and time management. This was a return to the original issues that are still very present and as such require innovative techniques.

In 2012, GISEH crossed the Atlantic and held its 6th conference in Quebec City at the *Centre Interuniversitaire de Recherche sur les Résaux d'Entreprise, la Logistique et le Transport* (CIRRELT). New techniques such as lean or risk management were widely discussed in areas ranging from hospitals to home care and general medicine. A total of 147 participants, including 67 hospital staff, came to listen to 70 presentations. The journey to the New World was a success.

The 7th GISEH conference took place in Liège in the summer of 2014, at the *Centre Hospitalier Universitaire de Sart Tilman*; it generated the highest turnout with 222 speakers. The theme for GISEH 2014, organized, run and supported by Liégeois hospitals was: "The Hospital: A Company Like Any Other?". An exciting and particularly topical subject in 2014, due to the requirement for all healthcare establishments and organizations to ensure a certain level and quality of service, while at the same time guaranteeing cost control. Engineering of healthcare systems, management of care systems, information systems, organizational development and knowledge management brought together the various presentations and generated numerous discussions.

Having crossed the Atlantic, the next international destination was the Mediterranean, and so the 8th GISEH conference came to Casablanca in the summer of 2016. It was hosted at the *Université Mohammed VI des Sciences de la Santé* and organized under the theme, "The Hospital and the Territorialization of Health: Transversality as a Key Factor of Sustainable Performance". It brought together 167 participants eager to discuss different health systems and multiple health situations. The French-speaking community of GISEH was thus fully established and served.

The 9th GISEH was organized in the summer of 2018 at the *Hôpitaux Universitaires de Genève*. The aim of GISEH 2018 was to focus on the performance of health systems, networks and institutions. Its objectives were to take stock of the situation, identify the causes of the problems and investigate the avenues and mechanisms that could be employed to improve the performance of health systems, networks and institutions. 260 participants promoted discussion on these themes through 76 presentations.

In 2020 the world was faced with a pandemic that led governments to confine over half of the human population. The *Université Polytechnique Hauts-de-France* continued to host the 10th GISEH, despite the travel constraints imposed by the health situation, by conducting the event through videoconferences. The theme for GISEH 2020 was, "Towards Innovative Health and Healthcare Institutions, Integrated in their Environments and Performance". One of the objectives was to study the integration of the hospital into healthcare and prevention approaches. There was also a focus on the situation of vulnerable people: children, the elderly, people with disabilities, people with cancer, etc. Thirty-five presentations were delivered despite the Covid-19 pandemic.

Thus far, 10 GISEH conferences have been held in French-speaking countries over the past 18 years. Academics and hospital staff, driven by the social, economic and environmental efficiency of essential human systems working towards the well-being of humanity, will have shared their ideas, built projects, put their solutions into practice and built common skills. At the ripe age of 63, I am leaving for the militant world of mutual insurance companies in healthcare. I leave the GISEH conferences in the capable hands of Philippe Wieser and Sondès Chaabane, two friends who have already made invaluable contributions to the success of these conferences.

Alain GUINET
Emeritus Professor
Chairman of the GISEH Steering Committee, 2003–2020
October 2021

Preface

Healthcare institutions will evolve towards becoming more innovative institutions by pursuing defined paths that consider risk factors and the collective and individual context of patients. They will take advantage of information technologies, scientific methods and mass data to prevent, anticipate, monitor and follow developments in public health, in order to intervene at the right time with the right tools. They will focus on people, be it the patient, the citizen or the caregivers by providing a high-performance health environment that meets safety, quality and productivity requirements.

The theme of this book centers around the engineering and management of healthcare and healthcare institutions, with the aim of making them agile and integrated into their environments. The book thus deals with the "hospital" system and the path to good health: issues, prevention approaches, data/IT, organizational innovations and recent technological solutions. It also opens up new opportunities for improving hospital systems with advances in artificial intelligence, information systems and service robotics.

The current context of the Covid-19 pandemic that we have been experiencing since early 2020 has only confirmed this need for openness, modernization and innovation in our healthcare systems. This crisis has shown us that we are vulnerable, that everyone is affected by these public health issues and that these can only be resolved through a collective and global effort. So, one wonders, what is the role of the hospital? Does it wait for a request for care? It is clear that the hospital cannot take care of everything and yet it should pay attention to everything. Our motivation for this book is to present scientific work that will allow our hospitals to evolve into innovative hospitals, open to their environment and efficient where health is concerned, not only to deliver care but also allowing citizens to prevent diseases and put their health at the heart of their priorities.

This book is presented in three different parts, each composed of five chapters that have been written by health professionals, researchers in science and technology, as well as in the human and social sciences from different French-speaking countries. The first part presents the various works that have been addressed optimization and simulation in healthcare systems. This research shows the potential and the opportunities offered by these techniques to support institutions in their management and organization of care methods. The second part focuses on digital and electronic technologies with an emphasis on artificial intelligence methods, allowing for the intelligent use of data or even robotization in the integration of technologies our healthcare offers, the working conditions of our caregivers or the assistance being afforded to fragile and vulnerable people. These first two parts highlight opportunities for innovative organizations and better management, as well as the threats related to changes in the daily life and practices of our institutions. The third part of the book therefore responds to the problems of change management and the impacts on our practices, our organizations and our management methods.

Sondès CHAABANE
October 2021

PART 1

Optimization and Simulation of Healthcare Systems

Summary of Contributions – Part 1

Towards a Prototype for the Strategic Recomputing of Schedules in Home Care Services, *by Cléa MARTINEZ, Maria DI MASCOLO, Marie-Laure ESPINOUSE and Jérôme RADUREAU.*

Home care is an alternative to traditional hospitalization to cope with aging populations and the increase in the number of vulnerable people whilst ensuring a good quality of life for patients. Even though these structures are developing more and more, the planning of their activities remains manual and can be time-consuming and exceedingly complex on a large scale. It is therefore essential to have effective solutions for planning interventions with an update mechanism to compensate for unforeseen events. This contribution therefore offers a decision support tool to solve the problem of long-term re-scheduling in the home care sector. A weekly planning update prototype was developed to meet a need expressed by a home care company operating in Auvergne Rhône-Alpes: Adomni-Quemera.

Home Healthcare Scheduling Activities, *by Rym BEN BACHOUCH JACQUIN and Jihene TOUNSI.*

This chapter examines the problem of planning rounds in hospitalization at home (HaH) by taking into account uncertainties and integrating dynamic re-scheduling. The authors propose an approach based on a genetic algorithm which considers re-scheduling in real time to resolve any conflicts that may arise as a result of unforeseen disruptions which may occur. This approach takes place in two phases. The first phase is carried out "offline", making it possible to establish the schedules of the nursing staff. The second phase is "online", making it possible to manage unforeseen events in real time, such as the absence of staff and delays in care. In the disrupted context, a new schedule is generated in order to cope with the disruption. The results obtained show the efficiency and robustness of the proposed approach with rapid computation time.

Optimal Sizing of an Automated Dispensing Cabinet under Adjacency Constraints, *by Khalid HACHEMI, Didier GOURC and François MARMIER.*

This contribution focuses on the dispensing phase of the medication circuit. This phase corresponds to the validation of the prescription, preparation and delivery of the medication. The main objective of the study is to minimize the errors that occur during this phase and, more specifically, in the case of automated dispensation cabinets. Such errors can occur when the cabinet is filled with the wrong product in the wrong place resulting in the wrong medication being delivered to the patient. To resolve this problem, the authors propose an algebraic model for the calculation of boundary conditions necessary for the allocation of medications to different compartments of a cabinet. This method must ensure that certain products are not placed in neighboring compartments due to the risk of confusion, which may lead to distribution errors, for example, medicinal products having a similar appearance, nomenclature or dosage. A modeling of the maximum permissive target problem (MPTP) has been proposed, as well as its resolution through a real-world digital application.

Validation of an Automated and Targeted Pharmaceutical Analysis Tool at the CHU de Liège, *by Sophie STREEL, Nathalie MAES, Véronique GONCETTE, Laurence SEIDEL, Denis MENAGER, Adelin ALBERT, Philippe KOLH and Didier MAESEN.*

This next contribution also looks at the medication flow, which can be a major challenge for a hospital. This flow is a complex and multidisciplinary process, which includes the clinical pathways (prescription, distribution, administration) and logistics (supply, transport, storage). The computerization of the medication flow at the "CHU de Liège" is widely implemented. This study describes how an automated and targeted pharmaceutical analysis tool was built, implemented and evaluated at the "CHU de Liège". The objective of this tool is to provide reliable and solid support to pharmacists for the verification of prescriptions so as to optimize and meet the hospital's accreditation criteria. Various pharmaceutical validation algorithms were thus constructed, and the computer validation tool was developed and tested on these bases which generated very encouraging results.

Simulation of Countermeasures in the Face of Covid-19 Using a Linear Compartmental Model, *by Alain GUINET.*

Since the start of 2020, the whole world has been confronted by a pandemic, which led to the confinement of over half of the world's inhabitants. We are disarmed in the face of the coronavirus (SARS-CoV-2), and containment seems to be the only countermeasure capable of containing the pandemic despite the consequential economic cost. This chapter presents a simulation of the epidemic based on the SIR (Susceptible–Infected–Recovered) model, which is known as a compartmental model in epidemiology. This simulation makes it possible to calculate, by period, the people at different stages of the disease, receiving different medical treatment, and to propagate the flows of people between the states by period. A discrete representation of the SIR model over a horizon of daily periods was used. The results showed the effectiveness of the health countermeasure chosen by half of the world's countries to deal with the Covid-19 pandemic. Containment of the population seems to be a well-suited action in the absence of an efficient treatment, such as viral treatment or a vaccine.

1

Towards a Prototype for the Strategic Recomputing of Schedules in Home Care Services

1.1. Introduction

Home healthcare agencies are an alternative to standard medical or paramedical organizations, providing services directly to the beneficiary's home. The aging of Western populations is accompanied by an increase in the number of vulnerable people and an explosion in demand for home healthcare and associated services (Guinet 2014), to which the organizations concerned must adapt. Service routing and scheduling is usually done by hand by experienced employees but this is time-consuming and extremely complex on a large scale. The design of decision support tools is becoming essential to automate the routing and scheduling process and build schedules that are satisfactory for the employer, the careworkers and the beneficiaries.

Having effective solutions to plan interventions is unfortunately not always sufficient to meet the challenge of routing and scheduling in the home care sector. Indeed, many eventualities can make a theoretically optimal schedule unfeasible. It is thus necessary to update the schedules to compensate for these unforeseen events. We are particularly interested in changes in the configuration of staff and beneficiaries of a home healthcare organization. Over the weeks, a beneficiary's state of health can deteriorate, which in turn leads to changes in their needs and therefore in the services required, or even bidding farewell to the organization in the event they require hospitalization, for example. When beneficiaries leave, the

---

Chapter written by Cléa MARTINEZ, Maria DI MASCOLO, Marie-Laure ESPINOUSE and Jérôme RADUREAU.

establishment can, if the number of careworkers is high enough, accept new beneficiaries who will have to be included in the schedules. Likewise, there is a high turnover of staff because the careworkers are often subjected to difficult, stressful working conditions.

From a strategic, decision-making point of view, it would be inappropriate to recalculate optimal routes every time the schedules are disrupted. In a context where the human aspect is essential, it is necessary to take into account the schedule in progress, the assignments of careworkers or even the start time of the interventions, in order to satisfactorily reconstruct disrupted routes. Indeed, continuity is a key factor in patient satisfaction. Consequently continuity of care constraints must be respected by, on the one hand, keeping fixed start and end times (these are also defined contractually) and on the other hand, always assigning the same group of careworkers to the same patients. In order not to aggravate these instabilities, it is also crucial to take careworker satisfaction into account. Schedules that are not satisfactory for the staff increase staff turnover, which impacts the company's quality of service. In a field where competition is increasingly fierce (Béguin 2018), providing good working conditions is not only a central argument for recruiting qualified careworkers but it also plays a decisive role in limiting turnover.

It is important to note that updating long-term schedules consists of creating new sustainable weekly or monthly schedules, in line with changes to staff and beneficiaries, while short-term rescheduling instead aims to provide a quick fix to the problem; for example, a daily schedule compromised by a one-off disruption, such as the sudden absence of a worker for a day.

In this chapter, we present a prototype developed to respond to a long-term weekly rerouting and rescheduling problem encountered by a home care services company operating in Auvergne Rhône-Alpes, France: Adomni-Quemera. We first offer a brief review of existing work on this theme in the literature, followed by a more specific description of the problem under consideration. In section 1.4, we briefly advance our resolution strategy, before presenting the prototype developed to propose solutions in a practical setting in section 1.5. The experiments carried out on real data are detailed in section 1.6. Finally, we approach avenues of research for future work in section 1.7.

1.2. Literature review

The Home Health Care Routing and Scheduling Problem (HHCRSP), i.e. the problem of planning home care routes, appears for the first time – to our knowledge – in 1997 in the article by Begur *et al.* (1997). Their method is based on adaptations of heuristics derived from algorithms for solving vehicle routing problems (VRP); in particular the classical methods developed in Clarke and Wright (1964) and Lin and Kernighan (1973). The modeling of the HHCRSP as a variant of the VRP is quite classic and Cheng and Rich (1998) were the first to adapt it to mixed-integer linear programming. They model the problem through a multi-depot vehicle routing problem (MDVRP) with multiple time windows, over a single-period horizon. The goal is to minimize overtime and tests are conducted on small case studies, made up of 4 nurses and 10 patients.

Since then, much research has focused on solving such problems, as they constitute a topical issue, both in practice and in the field of research with real scientific obstacles. For further details, the reader can refer to recent literature reviews: Cissé *et al.* (2017), Fikar and Hirsch (2017), Grieco *et al.* (2020) and Di Mascolo *et al.* (2021).

The problem is NP-hard, and thus difficult to solve in practice due to the presence of numerous business and industry-specific constraints, which are often treated with metaheuristics (Decerle *et al.* 2018) or with decomposition methods, such as the approach developed in the prototype presented here. In Grenouilleau *et al.* (2017), the authors propose a two-step algorithm to solve the routing and scheduling problem with minimization of overtime, staff qualification constraints and the possibility of not providing all the services requested. An LNS algorithm makes it possible to generate feasible routes, then a set partitioning model whose linear relaxation is repaired through a constructive heuristic, making it possible to select the routes that constitute the final schedule. In Fikar and Hirsch (2015), identification of potential routes precedes the overall scheduling optimization phase. The problem can also be broken down into a first step of assigning services to careworkers, then solving a traveling salesperson (TSP) problem for each of them. Issaoui *et al.* (2015) add a third step to this decomposition, in which they improve the routes obtained using a heuristic.

Most of the time, the objectives studied relate to the economic aspects of the problem, namely cost minimization (Fathollahi-Fard *et al.* 2019). However, there is also a particular interest in patient satisfaction (Mosquera *et al.* 2019). Careworker satisfaction, which is rarely studied, mainly consists of balancing the workload of careworkers (Cappanera and Scutellà 2014). The three stakeholders of the problem, namely the careworkers, the beneficiaries and the employer of the organization, generally have divergent interests and objectives. In Carello *et al.* (2018), a linear program, with several objective functions integrated into a threshold method, makes it possible to establish a compromise between all the stakeholders of the problem.

While the research cited above addresses the problem of static scheduling, it should be noted that in the home healthcare industry, it is rare to be able to maintain a functional schedule over a long period. Indeed, the instability inherent in the health sector quickly makes scheduling obsolete or not suited in the dynamic aspects of the problem (Cappanera *et al.* 2018).

In Heching *et al.* (2019), a Benders decomposition is used to accurately solve the problem of re-scheduling following the departure or arrival of patients. The first step is to solve an assignment problem with a mixed linear program. Next, a constraint programming model is used to plan the routes. The objective is to maximize the number of patients visited over a weekly period while respecting continuity constraints. In Nickel *et al.* (2012), the re-scheduling problem is solved by integrating new patients into the system with an insertion heuristic, then improving the solution with an LNS-type algorithm. The evolution of the patient population is considered in these two articles, while the composition of the staff remains unchanged.

In the literature, a wide range of constraints and objectives have been considered. However, much of the work remains theoretical and does not make it possible to deal with actual cases or to offer operational solutions given that, for example, legal constraints are often only partially addressed. In Szander *et al.* (2018), the authors want to reduce this gap between theoretical research and real-life situations through a case study of a home care center in Hungary, where the appointment times are fixed, and the objective is to minimize travel costs while maximizing beneficiary satisfaction through an MILP. In Gomes and Ramos (2019), the authors deal with a re-scheduling problem with the constraints of non-continuity of care that are not very common in the literature but which stem from actual cases encountered in Portugal: a non-profit organization and a Catholic parish where part of their mission is home help. Using different mixed linear programs, they are developing a multi-objective approach that aims to reduce travel times while minimizing the disruption associated with the departure and arrival of new patients. Once again, careworker changes are not considered here.

Thus, more and more works are interested in actual cases, even though their applied aspect is often limited to experiments on real data. Nevertheless, a few methods developed in direct relation with actors in the sector have made it possible to develop prototypes that can be used in practice and even software that is now deployed in practice. To the best of our knowledge, the first decision support system for this type of problem was proposed by Begur *et al.* (1997). An optimization module for the routing phase is integrated into a geographic information system that allows us to view routes. The LAPS CARE tool (Eveborn *et al.* 2006), now used in care units in Sweden, makes it possible to plan routes according to patient preferences and Swedish regulations. The proposed routes do not necessarily satisfy all the constraints and must be modified by the users when necessary. However, the scheduling task is made easier through the use of this tool, especially when it comes to quickly re-optimizing routes to deal with a last-minute, unforeseen event. More recently, a decision support system was created to support the Ottawa Hospital in its setup for home dialysis (Kandakoglu *et al.* 2020). Schedules are set by the day and last-minute disruptions are managed with the help of "floating" nurses who can act as replacements at a moment's notice.

Here, we are interested in a real-world scenario that includes more constraints than most of the work in the literature, as we consider almost all of the constraints arising from French national collective agreements (lunch breaks, work shifts, effective working time). We pay particular attention to the continuity of care, which constitutes a real scientific challenge. We consider the variations in beneficiaries as well as in the staff, and consider updating schedules on a strategic level, while most of the work in the literature is concerned with managing disruptions in the shorter term. Our aim is to propose solutions applicable in practice which therefore respect both the legislation and several rules of use and internal functioning of the organization with which we collaborate. We present a prototype whose objective is to allow the decision-makers to generate new schedules themselves, to keep the database up-to-date as careworkers and beneficiaries evolve. It should be noted that we find optimal solutions for real-size instances (up to 92 beneficiaries and 337 services).

1.3. Description of the problem

We consider the case of a home care organization that employs careworkers characterized by different levels of qualifications, specific time availability and a contractual and individualized monthly work volume. The organization plans its routes to provide a set of services required by a set of beneficiaries who need careworkers with different qualifications.

We assume that a schedule has already been established but has become obsolete due to changes in staff or beneficiaries. We consider the cases where one or more beneficiaries and/or careworkers leave the organization and where new beneficiaries and/or careworkers must instead be integrated into the schedules.

1.3.1. *Constraints*

New routes should be designed so that all services are provided while respecting constraints that we have divided into several categories: continuity constraints, legal constraints and constraints arising from the field.

1.3.1.1. *Continuity constraints*

Two types of continuity constraints are considered: time continuity constraints and human continuity constraints. These constraints are characteristic elements of the routing and scheduling update.

We must respect the continuity of the schedule by keeping the start and end times unchanged from those set initially. In our case study, these start and end times are indeed contractual and cannot be called into question for each change in the schedule.

Next, we must respect so-called "human" continuity constraints. We define a continuity rate for each beneficiary, depending on the number of careworkers they know and the maximum number of different careworkers they can tolerate. Depending on the value of this rate, the intervention of employees still unknown to the beneficiary may be authorized. This makes it possible both to integrate new arrivals into the schedules and to compensate for the departure of careworkers.

To our knowledge, the constraints of time continuity are rarely studied in the literature, if at all. As for the constraints of human continuity, they represent a scientific challenge.

1.3.1.2. *Legal constraints*

These constraints result from French collective agreements (Legifrance 2012).

This involves limiting the amplitude of a work day, the effective working time of a day, a week, and of a month, guaranteeing breaks, in particular the lunch break, and prohibiting too many breaks within a single day and, more specifically, long breaks.

By amplitude we refer to the total duration of a work day, except for the first and last trip of the day. The waiting time under the collective agreements corresponds to the time not worked that is less than 15 minutes between two successive interventions. As for the effective working time, this is the total duration of the services performed during the day with waiting times strictly less than 15 minutes between two services and travel times, except the first and last visit of the route. We make sure that each careworker has a lunch break and takes a break when working for longer than 6 hours at a time.

Finally, a careworker must have the necessary qualifications to provide a service and overqualified work is allowed.

1.3.1.3. *Internal policies*

Some constraints are internal policies inherent in the home care industry or those specific to the organization in which we are interested. We build quarter-hour schedules, for obvious practical reasons. We allow for overtime but within a limit of 20% of the contractual hourly volume of the careworker concerned. It is possible to run two services consecutively with overlapping schedules if the duration of this overlap (including travel time) does not exceed 10 minutes. Finally, when the schedule is carried out for a week, the monthly contractual hourly volume is reduced to a weekly volume by dividing the monthly volume by 4.33.

1.3.2. *Objective function*

The goal is to minimize the total waiting time induced by the schedule, i.e., the sum of all the careworker waiting times over the planning horizon. As we want to provide satisfactory schedules for careworkers, we count the waiting times as the sum of all the time not worked that is less than 90 minutes between two successive interventions, not counting the travel times. Indeed, when careworkers have an inactivity time of more than 90 minutes, we consider that they can take advantage of this period to conduct personal activities.

1.4. Resolution method

Our resolution method is an exact method that is based on a decomposition of the problem into two sub-problems: the generation of the set of admissible daily routes and then the selection of a set of daily routes to carry out a weekly schedule (or possibly a monthly schedule).

In a previous article (Martinez *et al.* 2019), we proposed an algorithm which allowed us to solve a similar theoretical problem. In the prototype presented here, we have adapted it in order to take into account all the routing and scheduling constraints and cover all the perturbations considered, and not just the departure of beneficiaries. We are not focusing here on the developed method but rather on its implementation and its integration into the prototype.

1.4.1. *Route generation*

We start by generating a set of graphs, one for each day and careworker, in order to represent our problem. For a particular graph, a set of vertices represents the set of services that could be provided by this careworker, that is, the services for which he or she is qualified, whose start and end times correspond to their availability, and for which the beneficiary is compatible with the continuity constraints of the problem. To this set of vertices, we add two fictitious services representing the start and end points of a route.

We then create arcs between all the pairs of services which could be performed consecutively by the same careworker. It is thus a matter of ensuring that the start and end times of the two services are compatible, in particular with regard to the travel time between the homes of the two beneficiaries concerned.

A route from the source to the sink thus represents a sequence of compatible services, i.e., a daily route. This route will be said to be admissible if it respects all the daily legal constraints. By constructing the graph, we have already made sure that the constraints of continuity and qualifications are respected.

We weight each arc by the travel time between the two homes of the beneficiaries concerned, the duration of the arc's first service and the waiting time between the two services, in terms of the collective agreements. If we generate a route from the source to the sink by limiting its length, then we can control the amplitude, the effective working time and the waiting time of the route to which it corresponds. By adapting the algorithm proposed in Rizzi *et al.* (2015), we can efficiently compute all the admissible daily routes for a careworker on a given day.

1.4.2. *Route selection*

Once all the routes have been generated, we need to assign one route per careworker per day, to ensure that the weekly and/or monthly legal constraints are respected and that the overall waiting time of the careworkers is minimal. For this purpose, we use a linear integer program to solve this set partitioning problem. We add constraints to ensure that the weekly (or monthly) working regulations defined in the French collective agreements are respected, as well as the human continuity constraints.

1.5. Presentation of the prototype

The optimization module described above was developed in Java. We have also developed a basic graphical interface in Excel, which also contains all the data relating to the beneficiaries and the staff of the home care service organization under consideration, as well as the parameters resulting from our case study, which are necessary for the execution of the algorithm. The interface provided allows the user to make changes to the database and software settings and then generate routes.

Thanks to dedicated forms, the user can add new beneficiaries or careworkers, modify those who are already entered in the database or delete them. The distance and travel time calculations between beneficiaries are then calculated automatically from the addresses entered, using the data provided by Google Maps via its geolocation API.

The parameters relating to the rules that are the result of the collective agreements and internal policies of our applied case can also be modified, as well as the sectorization of the territory covered by the company.

The user provides a previously designed, initial schedule. From the database updated with the latest developments in staff and beneficiaries, the prototype recalculates the routes and generates an Excel file with the list of changes that compares to the initial schedule that was supplied as an input. The decision-maker will thus have the list of reassigned interventions with their date, their start and end times (unchanged since they are contractually fixed), the name of the beneficiary and the name of the newly assigned careworker.

1.6. Tests and results

We conduct our tests across several geographic areas in which Adomni-Quemera operates. We start from the initial weekly schedules established in August 2019 and update this schedule to match the October 2019 beneficiary and stakeholder population, which had changed since August. The results are given in Table 1.1. Each instance is characterized by its number of current beneficiaries, its number of current careworkers and the number of services required for the week. In the "Beneficiary variation" column (resp. "Careworker variation"), we specify the number of changes in the beneficiaries (resp. careworkers) compared to when the initial planning was established. Thus, "+1/-2" means that one person has integrated the organization and that two people have left. Next, we indicate the sum of the waiting times and travel times for all careworkers over the whole week. Finally, we indicate the execution time of the algorithm.

The tests were carried out on a machine with the following characteristics: Intel RCoreTMi5-7440HQ CPU 2.80GHz with 16GB of RAM. The optimization algorithm was developed in Java, and we used CPLEX to solve the PLNE. On each of the instances processed, we have variation in beneficiaries and/or careworkers, for which it should be noted that the overall hourly volume of work and the overall hourly volume of services requested remains similar to those provided in the initial schedule.

Due to the method being exact, we found the optimal solution for each of the proposed instances, that is, the solution that minimizes the overall waiting time of the careworkers. Execution times are very fast (at worst, in the order of a minute on the instances tested). Note that minimizing waiting times produces solutions with very low travel times, except for two instances (4 and 7). Since *Instance 7* is the largest in terms of the number of careworkers, the average travel times per careworker are in fact no longer than for the other instances. We can compare the results with *Instance 6*, which has more careworkers but almost half as many services. The routes are far less busy, involving less travel and therefore less travel time. For *Instance 4*, because the associated sector is geographically larger, the longer travel times are not surprising. However, as we have no constraints or objectives of minimizing travel times, it is not excluded that there is a solution with equivalent waiting times but shorter travel times.

We can notice that *Instances 5* and *6* have a similar number of services. As the variations of careworkers are much greater in *Instance 6*, the continuity constraints are harder to respect and the graphs constructed through our method are denser. This explains the difference in execution times.

Note also that waiting times greater than 90 minutes are not counted. Therefore, it is possible that the routes produced are fragmented, which implies a long amplitude. While a long break in the day is not disruptive, it is not desirable, and as such having a compact route is also a criterion of staff satisfaction.

Instance	Number of beneficiaries	Number of careworkers	Number of services	Beneficiary variations	Careworkers variations	Waiting time (h)	Travel time (h)	Execution time (s)
1	3	4	56	–	+1/-1	4. 2	3. 8	2. 2
2	11	5	85	+0/-1	+2/-3	4. 69	6. 49	2. 1
3	18	6	95	+2/-4	–	8. 41	5. 7	7. 6
4	26	8	156	+2/-7	+2/-3	1. 5	19.3	40.6
5	26	11	179	+6/-5	+2/-2	7. 15	6. 4	30.13
6	40	18	191	+8/-11	+8/-6	5. 83	1. 83	65.8
7	92	15	337	+7/-10	+3/-5	12. 0	21.3	101

Table 1.1. *Numerical results*

1.7. Conclusion and perspectives

We have developed a method that solves real-world problems by taking into account the legal constraints resulting from French national collective agreements, internal policies specific to our case study, as well as changes to beneficiaries and staff. The objective of minimizing waiting times is to improve the working conditions of staff in order to limit turnover. These waiting times are calculated using Adomni-Quemera's definition. However, while some periods of inactivity are perceived by careworkers as wasted time, others are viewed as real breaks and can be appreciated by staff. Proposing a new definition of waiting times, based on the experiences of careworkers, could result in new schedules that are even more satisfactory and adapted to each person. We can also consider a multi-objective approach which would also make it possible to limit the travel time and/or the amplitudes of the work shifts, which do not always go hand in hand with the minimization of waiting times.

Time constraints turn out to be a scientific obstacle and can contribute to a substantial degradation of the schedule. A tool identifying the most impinging time constraints would make it possible to determine the services for which it would be advantageous to renegotiate the contractual hours with the beneficiaries.

The proposed method is adapted to changes in the composition of staff and beneficiaries and to the strategic update; however, it is not necessarily adequate in the event of a one-off absence. Indeed, if a worker is temporarily unavailable, the organization does not always have a careworker available who is qualified to replace them at short notice. It is therefore necessary to overload the other careworkers and potentially shift the appointment times so as to be able to obtain a feasible solution. Respecting the continuity of care constraints becomes very restrictive and is no longer necessarily relevant. Moreover, as these absences are often unexpected, it is difficult in practice to upset the whole schedule at the last minute. Thus, it would be interesting to adapt our approach to the management of daily eventualities, by relaxing the constraints of continuity and by considering stability from a new angle: no longer that of continuity of care, but rather with the objective of impacting as few routes as possible, in order to meet operational requirements in the field.

1.8. References

Béguin, F. (2018). Le nombre de candidats aux écoles d'aides-soignants en baisse. *Le Monde* [Online]. Available at: https://www.lemonde.fr/sante/article/2018/05/11/le-nombre-de-candidats-aux-ecoles-d-aides-soignants-en-baisse_5297453_1651302.html.

Begur, S.V., Miller, D.M., Weaver, J.R. (1997). An integrated spatial DSS for scheduling and routing home-health-care nurses. *Interfaces*, 27, 35–48.

Cappanera, P. and Scutellà, M.G. (2014). Joint assignment, scheduling, and routing models to home care optimization: A pattern-based approach. *Transportation Science*, 49, 830–852.

Cappanera, P., Scutellà, M.G., Nervi, F., Galli, L. (2018). Demand uncertainty in robust home care optimization. *Omega*, 80, 95–110.

Carello, G., Lanzarone, E., Mattia, S. (2018). Trade-off between stakeholders' goals in the home care nurse-to-patient assignment problem. *Operations Research for Health Care*, 16, 29–40.

Cheng, E. and Rich, J.L. (1998). A home health care routing and scheduling problem. Technical report [Online]. Available at: https://scholarship.rice.edu/handle/1911/101899.

Cissé, M., Yalçındağ, S., Kergosien, Y., Şahin, E., Lenté, C., Matta, A. (2017). OR problems related to home health care: A review of relevant routing and scheduling problems. *Operations Research for Health Care*, 13–14, 1–22.

Clarke, G. and Wright, J.W. (1964). Scheduling of vehicles from a central depot to a number of delivery points. *Operations Research*, 12, 568–581.

Decerle, J., Grunder, O., Hajjam El Hassani, A., Barakat, O. (2018). A memetic algorithm for a home health care routing and scheduling problem. *Operations Research for Health Care*, 16, 59–71.

Di Mascolo, M., Martinez, C., Espinouse, M.L. (2021). Routing and scheduling in home health care: A literature survey and bibliometric analysis. *Computers & Industrial Engineering*, 158, 107255.

Eveborn, P., Flisberg, P., Rönnqvist, M. (2006). LAPS CARE: An operational system for staff planning of home care. *European Journal of Operational Research*, 171(3), 962–976.

Fathollahi-Fard, A.M., Hajiaghaei-Keshteli, M., Mirjalili, S. (2019). A set of efficient heuristics for a home healthcare problem. *Neural Computing and Applications*, 32, 6185–6205.

Fikar, C. and Hirsch, P. (2015). A matheuristic for routing real-world home service transport systems facilitating walking. *Journal of Cleaner Production*, 105, 300–310.

Fikar, C. and Hirsch, P. (2017). Home health care routing and scheduling: A review. *Computers & Operations Research*, 77, 86–95.

Gomes, M.I. and Ramos, T.R.P. (2019). Modelling and (re-)planning periodic home social care services with loyalty and non-loyalty features. *European Journal of Operational Research*, 277, 284–299.

Grenouilleau, F., Legrain, A., Lahrichi, N., Rousseau, L.-M. (2017). A set partitioning heuristic for the home health care routing and scheduling problem [Online]. Available at: http://www.cirrelt.ca/DocumentsTravail/CIRRELT-2017-70.pdf.

Grieco, L., Utley, M., Crowe, S. (2020). Operational research applied to decisions in home health care: A systematic literature review. *Journal of the Operational Research Society*, 1–32.

Guinet, A. (2014). Organisation des soins à domicile en Europe et Amérique du Nord. *Proceedings from the 10th Conférence francophone de modélisation, optimisation et simulation (MOSIM)*, Nancy, France.

Heching, A., Hooker, J.N., Kimura, R. (2019). A logic-based benders approach to home healthcare delivery. *Transportation Science*, 53, 510–522.

Issaoui, B., Zidi, I., Marcon, E., Ghedira, K. (2015). New multi-objective approach for the home care service problem based on scheduling algorithms and variable neighborhood descent. *Electronic Notes in Discrete Mathematics*, 47, 181–188.

Kandakoglu, A., Sauré, A., Michalowski, M., Aquino, M., Graham, J., McCormick, B. (2020). A decision support system for home dialysis visit scheduling and nurse routing. *Decision Support Systems*, 130, 113224.

Légifrance (2012). Convention collective nationale des entreprises de services à la personne du 20 septembre 2012 [Online]. Available at: https://www.legifrance.gouv.fr/affichIDCCArticle.do;jsessionid=1133A88F6CF2A4DE8D36FD10BF728C52.tplgfr42s_1?idArticle=KALIARTI000026943205&cidTexte=KALITEXT000026943I9.

Lin, S. and Kernighan, B.W. (1973). An effective heuristic algorithm for the traveling-salesman problem. *Operations Research*, 21, 498–516.

Martinez, C., Espinouse, M.-L., Di Mascolo, M. (2019). Re-planning in home healthcare: A decomposition approach to minimize idle times for workers while ensuring continuity of care. *Proceedings of the IFAC Conference on Manufacturing Modeling, Management and Control*, Berlin, Germany.

Mosquera, F., Smet, P., Vanden Berghe, G. (2019). Flexible home care scheduling. *Omega*, 83, 80–95.

Nickel, S., Schröder, M., Steeg, J. (2012). Mid-term and short-term planning support for home health care services. *European Journal of Operational Research*, 219, 574–587.

Rizzi, R., Sacomoto, G., Sagot, M.-F. (2015). Efficiently listing bounded length *st*-paths. In *Combinatorial Algorithms, Lecture Notes in Computer Science*, Jan, K., Miller, M., Froncek, D. (eds). Springer, Berlin.

Szander, N., Ros-McDonnell, L.B., Bogataj, M. (2018). A feasible nurse routing plan for the elderly: Quality and spatial trade-offs. In *Closing the Gap Between Practice and Research in Industrial Engineering, Lecture Notes in Management and Industrial Engineering*, Viles, E., Ormazábal, M., Lleó, A. (eds). Springer, Berlin.

2

Home Healthcare Scheduling Activities

2.1. Introduction

Home healthcare (HHC) is a field of research which, due to its complexity in terms of organization and diversity of players, not to mention in the medical and social specificities of patients, opens up several fields of investigation. We can identify the optimization challenges inherent to the management of the HHC structure, which in turn leads to significant research activity on problems concerning nurse rostering and drug deliveries. The optimization problem in HHC must take into account several constraints related to the organization of the structure, the patient, road traffic, emergencies, etc. The purpose is to ensure visits to patients according to their care plans. One of the major constraints in the organization of care is taking into account emergencies as well as uncertainties such as changes in the duration of care and also the disturbances caused by the external environment (road traffic, for example).

In this chapter, we present a solution for the HHC planning problem by integrating uncertainties and dynamic rescheduling. We first present a literature review with recent works that have focused on HHC planning. Section 2.3 focus on the proposed approach, which is based on a genetic algorithm with the consideration of real-time disturbances and uncertainties. Section 2.4 presents the experiments and the obtained results. We finish this chapter with a conclusion and some perspectives.

2.2. State of the art

The increase of the number of elderly people in France has led to a substantial increase in the demand for HHC services (e.g. home support structures, home hospitalization, etc.). This demand is due to two main causes:

Chapter written by Rym BEN BACHOUCH JACQUIN and Jihene TOUNSI.

– home care is less expensive for health insurance companies and helps to relieve congestion in hospitals;

– people who are still autonomous want to stay at home and benefit from HHC services (cleaning, reading, meal delivery, etc.).

HHC structures play an important role in the development of the silver economy and offer better well-being for elderly people. However, the organization of HHC is complex and difficult to control due to the multiplicity and diversity of players, their status (private or public), as well as their function (medical, paramedical, social, administrative). Moreover, each treatment is specific and must be personalized insofar as it relies on the patient's level of dependency.

HHC services require coordinated organization between all the stakeholders involved in the patient care plan. This coordination must take into account organizational and geographical constraints, working hours and constraints related to the patients (availability, preferences, activities of daily living, etc.).

Several constraints must be taken into account in HHC scheduling problems (Fikar and Hirsch 2017). Three classes of constraints have been identified: time constraints, assignment constraints and geographic constraints. The first class concerns the constraints associated with temporal relationships, that is, at what time the HHC service can take place or the time at which a caregiver can provide a service according to their schedule. Assignment constraints are linked to the relationships between caregivers and patients. They have a direct impact on the selection of the caregiver who is able and qualified to visit a patient. Finally, the last group of geographic constraints concern the location and the means of transport (Emiliano *et al.* 2017).

Planning the activities of HHC workers can be compared to the vehicle routing problem (VRP) or the traveling salesman problem (TSP) (Cissé *et al.* 2017). These problems have the same objectives and are subject to the same constraints but with specific features related to the types of clients and stakeholders. One of the main specificities in HHC planning activities is the constraints related to the patient for whom care must be provided. Indeed, there are different patient profiles according to their dependency level and the number/types of visits required.

Some studies have focused on chemotherapy, where the constraint of expiring drugs is a priority (Shahnejat-Busheir *et al.* 2019). In some cases, the structures employ full-time and part-time staff. We then try to ensure that each employee has their own assigned shift while adhering to work schedules. In addition, patient satisfaction remains the priority (Nasir *et al.* 2018; Di Mascolo *et al.* 2018) and penalties can be added if patient preferences are not respected (Nasir *et al.* 2015).

Therefore, continuity of care is a very important constraint (Hewitt *et al.* 2016; Lanzarone and Matta 2014; Wirnitzer *et al.* 2015). Other work (Cappanera 2013; Cardoso *et al.* 2015; David and Kim 2018) has focused on the workload distribution between caregivers in order to balance the workload and strenuousness. Each caregiver has a lunchtime break each day, which is a constraint for the schedule. We can consider a flexible lunchtime break that depends on visits in order to optimize the caregiver schedule (Xiao *et al.* 2018).

The problem of HHC scheduling consists of assigning caregivers to patients with the objective of satisfying the patient's care plan (Di Mascolo *et al.* 2017) and taking into account that some patients may need to have several visits during the day (Martinez *et al.* 2019). In some cases, we must also take into account the means of transport chosen by the provider (car or public transport) and sustainable development by, for example, the use of electric cars (Erdem and Koç 2019; Fathollahi-Fard *et al.* 2019). The vehicle fleet should also be synchronized with the caregiver's schedules and the shared visits (Nasir and Kuo 2020). In addition to these constraints, there are uncertainty problems linked to road traffic, personnel absence, etc. (Hewitt *et al.* 2016; Shi *et al.* 2017; Cappanera *et al.* 2018; Shi *et al.* 2019; Nikzad *et al.* 2020).

Home hospitalization is an area where, in some cases and for some patients, activities are interdependent. They may also require more than one careworker in the case of shared visits, for example (Redjem *et al.* 2011; Decerle *et al.* 2018, 2019). To solve this problem, some studies have created time slots for care. Caregivers are assigned to patients and time slots. Thus, an initial distribution between caregivers and time slots is established (Moussavi *et al.* 2019).

Several methods from operations research have been adapted to HHC problems (Brailsford and Vissers 2011) and especially to the planning problems that can be formulated as a Vehicle Routing Problem with Time Windows (Mutingi and Mbohwa 2013; Issaoui *et al.* 2015; Nasir *et al.* 2018; Xiao *et al.* 2018). Other works have used metaheuristics (Nickel *et al.* 2012; Grenouilleau *et al.* 2019, 2020; Nikzad *et al.* 2020), immune algorithms (Ben Hassen *et al.* 2019), genetic algorithms (Nasir and Kuo 2020), multi-agent systems (Widmer and Premm 2015, pp. 233–248; Marcon *et al.* 2017; Stojanova *et al.* 2017; Xie *et al.* 2017), ant colonies (Decerle *et al.* 2019), simulated annealing and tabu search (Shahnejat-Busheir *et al.* 2019) or even Markov chains (Koeleman *et al.* 2012).

HHC scheduling is a very important problem but rescheduling also remains a crucial challenge. The structures must cope with disruptions due to staff absences, the worsening of a patient's condition, variations in the care duration, etc. Mosquera *et al.* (2019) offer flexible durations of care and routes with a compromise between the number of treatments and the workloads of caregivers. We observe that few studies have addressed the rescheduling problem. In the following section, we present the proposed approach to address the HHC scheduling problem.

2.3. Description of the proposed approach

In this section, we describe the proposed solution to solve the HHC scheduling problem. The approach is based on two phases. The first is done "offline" and establishes the caregiver schedules. The second phase is done "online" and manages all unforeseen events, especially staff absences and change in care duration or travel time. In case of a disruption, the scheduler needs to regenerate all the schedules in real time. This approach is similar to the periodic repair approach proposed by Xie (2016). In the next section we detail the implementation of the "offline" and "online" phases.

2.3.1. *Home healthcare planning "offline phase"*

The HHC planning problem can be seen as an extension of the traveling salesman problem (TSP) or the vehicle routing problem (VRP) where we have a set of points to visit and a defined resource number. The objective of our approach is to minimize the travel cost of the medical staff, according to constraints related to the HHC structure, patient care plans and caregiver working hours.

In order to solve this problem, we use the genetic algorithm (GA) originally developed by Holland (1975). It is an evolutionary algorithm that maintains a population of candidate solutions for the problem studied and evolves it by iteratively applying a set of stochastic operators. This algorithm represents the dynamic behavior of our scheduling agent in an "offline" mode.

In Figure 2.1, we present the steps of the genetic algorithm to assign visits to caregivers and to subsequently generate the optimal routes. The three main operators of the proposed algorithm (reproduction, crossing and mutation) are applied on a random population in order to create a new generation. The route is evaluated and tested until the termination criterion, iteratively modified by GA operators, is met. The system examines whether an optimal solution is obtained, that is, whether the visits are assigned to caregivers and all constraints are respected (Vishnupriyan *et al.* 2008).

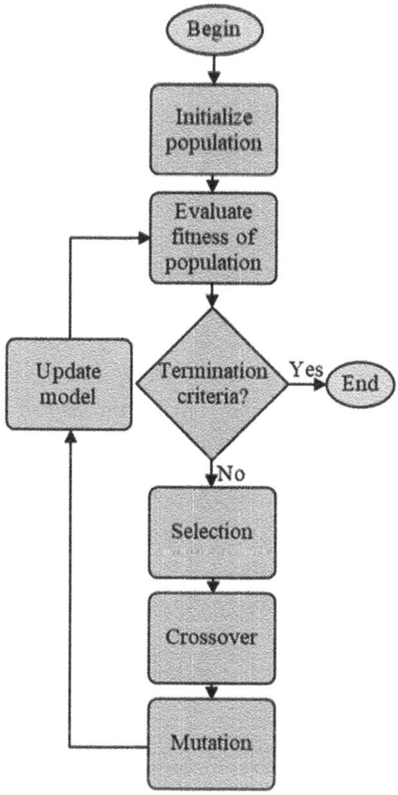

Figure 2.1. *Genetic algorithm (source: (Vishnupriyan* et al. *2008). For a color version of this figure, see www.iste.co.uk/chaabane/healthcare.zip*

Another extension of the genetic algorithm is the grouping genetic algorithm (GGA) initially proposed by Falkenauer (1992), which is suitable for solving grouping or classification problems. The general structure of the GGA is similar to the GA. The only difference lies in the internal mechanisms of the coding scheme and the implementation of the genetic operators. We present our solution based on the GGA and the methods chosen for each step.

GGA coding scheme. The structure of the genetic coding applied in this algorithm can strongly influence the performance of the GGA (Filho and Tiberti 2006; Mutingi and Mbohwa 2012). Mutingi and Mbohwa have developed a unique coding scheme that exploits the group structure for the scheduling problem. Let C = [1, n] be a chromosome representing a set of n patients who need to be visited by m caregivers. The purpose of this representation is to simplify the patient grouping across set C into m groups.

Population initialization. This step consists of creating a population of N elements, each with randomly generated DNA. DNA is created by randomly assigning patients to caregivers. A good technique might be to start by organizing the activities in ascending order of their starting times and, in some cases, to even organize them according to their duration. This procedure increases the likelihood that the initialization process will generate good solutions.

Fitness assessment. The fitness function tests the adequacy of the solution in relation with the problem being considered. Let (i, j) be a possible route, the caregiver starts from origin 0, which is generally the HHC structure, and visits the nodes $\{i, i+1, i+2, \ldots, j\text{-}1, j\}$. In our case, we have to calculate a score c_{ij} (equation [2.1]), thus calculating the sum of the distances traveled by the caregiver from their starting point, until they return to the HHC at the end of their schedules. Likewise, the fitness function must take into consideration time constraints, that is, the penalties incurred in the case of violating a patient's availability time window.

$$c_{ij} = v\left(d_{0,i+1} + \sum_{h=i+1}^{j-1} d_{h,h+1} + d_{j,0}\right) + k_e \sum_{i}^{j} \max(0, l_i - a_i) + k_l \sum_{i}^{j} \max(0, e_i - a_i) + Q_u \quad [2.1]$$

d_{ij} denotes the distances between two patients i and j; v represents the cost per distance traveled; k_e and k_l represent, respectively, the penalties when a caregiver arrives at the patient's home too early or too late; e_i and l_i denote the availability time window of patient i and a_i indicates the caregiver arrival time at the home of patient i. We have also integrated the variable Q_u into the fitness function to designate whether a care worker is qualified to perform a treatment or a visit or not. We considered a correlation between the caregiver qualification and the patient dependency level. The variable Q_u can be equal to 1 or 0 indicating, respectively, a qualified or unqualified caregiver.

Selection. Once the score has been calculated for the whole population, we can select the most adapted individuals to become parents. There are different approaches for the selection. In our case, we have chosen to apply a probabilistic method called "roulette wheel selection".

Crossing. This is a mechanism by which the selected chromosomes produce a new generation. This genetic operator will help us to explore the full range of possible solutions.

Mutation. Once the new chromosome is generated, we apply the mutation before adding the child to the next generation. Mutation consists of altering a gene in the generated chromosome. We include the new population in the old list and then we repeat from step 2.

Stop condition. The process is repeated until a maximum number of generations is reached. When looking for an optimal solution, many conditions are taken into account. A workload is limited to up to four patients for each caregiver, and patients are visited according to their availability windows.

2.3.2. *Rescheduling in online mode*

The routes generated by the offline algorithm may be subject to changes due to unforeseen events. In order to integrate a dynamic and reactive aspect to the proposed algorithm, we propose the management of in real time uncertainties related to caregiver availability or delay due to a change in activity duration. Caregivers should send notifications at the start and end of each visit through a dedicated mobile application. If they are late or unable to complete the assigned activity, they should immediately notify this to the planning officer. As a result, the scheduling agent executes the rescheduling algorithm (online) to reassign care to another available caregiver. The objective is to be able to carry out all the planned visits with the available caseworkers while respecting all the constraints shown in Figure 2.2.

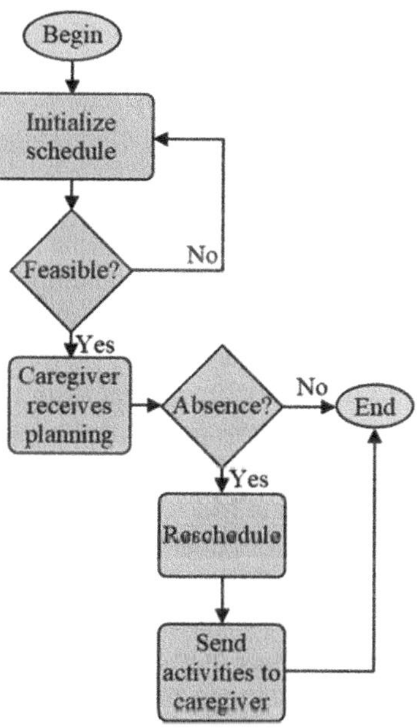

Figure 2.2. *Online rescheduling process. For a color version of this figure, see www.iste.co.uk/chaabane/healthcare.zip*

To ensure that the rescheduling step takes place in case of disruptions, the planning officer needs to know the availability of careworkers. The required information is provided by notifications from caregivers. The planning officer has all the necessary information about patients' preferences. When the new plan is generated, the agent sends it to the workers concerned after generating the new schedule (equation [2.2]).

$$< SA, MSA_k, V_m(t), TreatmentTime(V_m), PC, PS > \quad [2.2]$$

SA corresponds to the scheduling agent who is the request sender, MSA_k represents the care worker k with a modification on their schedule, $V_m(t)$ corresponds to the vector containing all the tasks t to be performed by MSA_k, TreatmentTime (V_m) corresponds to the duration of the treatment $V_m(t)$, PC refers to the geolocation coordinates of the patient and PS corresponds to the full patient features. When an MSA_k receives a new schedule, they must approve it by notifying the SA scheduling agent.

To conclude, we have chosen a modeling approach based on two phases. The first phase is establishing caregiver schedules in an offline mode. The second phase, dedicated to the management of disruptions, generates a new schedule in real time, that is, online. It consists of rescheduling the GGA algorithm several times, taking into consideration the available caregivers and the associated information known at the time of the rescheduling (the state of their current schedule and their geolocation).

2.4. Experiments and results

In order to ensure better patient care, we develop a platform that optimizes routes by taking into account the constraints related to patients and caregivers. The medical and coordination staff can thus communicate with each other and receive information on the patients treated and those still waiting for treatment. The platform is developed used for both offline planning and online rescheduling. It also allows the HHC schedule coordinator to record and consult the information needed. The main component of this platform is the genetic clustering algorithm. This algorithm communicates with Google Maps API to display the routes of caregivers as well as the geographical location of patients.

The algorithm assigns caregivers to patients based on availability, qualification and preference constraints. Patients are automatically identified on the map via their address, which is used for the calculation of the distances traveled. The routes are then determined according to the constraints. If a caregiver is absent or late, their status is updated and the routes are recalculated in order to take this information into account.

The results obtained from the route planning and calculation experiments are presented in Table 2.1. We tested the algorithm on examples ranging from 2 to 16 careworkers with 2 to 64 patients. The computation times remained quite fast; however, we noticed that as the number of patients and caregivers increases, the computation time becomes longer.

Number of caregivers	Number of patients	Computation time (s)
	2	1.58
2	4	3.27
	8	5.09
	4	7.43
4	8	10.60
	16	12.44
	8	13.80
8	16	14.38
	32	16.73
	16	18.62
16	32	20.01
	64	22.69

Table 2.1. *Results and experiments*

Number of disturbances	Number of reassigned visits per caregiver	Computation time (s)
	1	4.66–5.09
1	2	4.66–5.09
	3	4.66–5.09
	1	4.66–5.09
2	2	4.66–5.09
	3	4.66–5.09
	1	4.66–5.09
4	2	4.66–5.09
	3	4.70–5.36

Table 2.2. *Case of rescheduling with disruptions*

We also tested the rescheduling algorithm by adding disruptions represented by staff absences. The rescheduling phase can occur after the first route is calculated. Table 2.2 presents the results obtained when we have one to four disruptions. These visits are reassigned to other caregivers, and we find that each caregiver has one to three visits added to their initial schedule. Rescheduling is achieved in seconds. It is very efficient for the coordinator who needs a reactive system.

2.5. Conclusions and perspectives

In this chapter, we have focused on the HHC scheduling and rescheduling problems. We took into account the constraints related to the preferences, availabilities and dependency levels of patients as well as the qualifications and working hours of caregivers.

We have developed a genetic algorithm that calculates a schedule and also takes into account disruptions in real time. Re-planning makes it possible to reassign the unachieved activities in the case of an absence in a very short time (a few seconds). We were able to show the robustness and efficiency of our approach, which allows the scheduler manager to obtain all the schedule in few seconds, whether for the purposes of planning or rescheduling.

From the perspective of research, in future studies we will be able to integrate uncertainties related to the care duration as well as to take into account the rescheduling of other criteria, such as the absence of a patient at home or the development of their care condition.

2.6. References

Ben Hassen, H., Tounsi, J., Ben Bachouch, R. (2019). An artificial immune algorithm for HHC planning based on multi-agent system. *Procedia Computer Science*, 164, 251–256.

Braislford, S. and Vissers, J. (2011). OR in healthcare: A European perspective. *European Journal of Operational Research*, 212(2), 223–234.

Cappanera, P. (2013). Home care optimization: Impact of pattern generation policies on scheduling and routing decisions. *Electronic Notes in Discrete Mathematics*, 41, 53–60.

Cappanera, P., Scutella, M.G., Nervi, F., Galli, L. (2018). Demand uncertainty in robust home care optimization. *Omega*, 80, 95–110.

Cardoso, T., Oliveira, M.D., Barbosa-Povoa, A., Nickel, S. (2015). An integrated approach for planning a long-term care network with uncertainty, strategic policy and equity considerations. *European Journal of Operational Research*, 247, 321–334.

Cissé, M., Yalçindag, S., Kergosien, Y., Sahin, E., Lenté, C., Matta, A. (2017). OR problems related to home health care: A review of relevant routing and scheduling problems. *Operations Research for Health Care*, 13–14(C), 1–22.

David, G. and Kim, K.L. (2018). The effect of workforce assignment on performance: Evidence from home health care. *Journal of Health Economics*, 59, 26–45.

Decerle, J., Grunder, O., El Hassani, A.H., Barakat, O. (2018). A memetic algorithm for a home health care routing and scheduling problem. *Operations Research for Health Care*, 16, 59–71.

Decerle, J., Grunder, O., El Hassani, A.H., Barakat, O. (2019). A memetic algoritm for multi-objective optimization of the home health care problem. *Swarm and Evolutionary Computation*, 44, 712–727.

Di Mascolo, M., Espinouse, M.L., El Hajri, Z., (2017). Planning in home health care structures: A literature review. *IFAC PapersOnLine*, 50(1), 4656–4659.

Di Mascolo, M., Espinouse, M.L., Ait Haddadene, S.R. (2018). Taking patients' wishes into account for daily planning in the home health care context. *IFAC PapersOnLine*, 51(11), 1010–1015.

Emiliano, W., Telhada, J., Do Sameiro Carvalho, M. (2017). Home health care logistics planning: A review and framework. *Procedia Manufacturing*, 13, 848–955.

Erdem, M. and Koç, C. (2019). Analysis of electric vehicles in home health care routing problem. *Journal of Cleaner Production*, 234, 1471–1483.

Falkenauer, E. (1992). The grouping genetic algorithms – Widening the scope of the GAs. *Belgian Journal of Operations Research, Statistics and Computer Science*, 6, 79–102.

Fathollahi-Fard, A.M., Govindan, K., Hajiaghaei-Keshteli, M., Ahmadi, A. (2019). A green home health care supply chain: New modified simulated annealing algorithms. *Journal of Cleaner Production*, 240.

Fikar, C. and Hirsch, P. (2017). Home health care routing and scheduling: A review. *Computers and Operations Research*, 77, 86–95.

Filho, E.V.G. and Tiberti, A.J. (2006). A group genetic algorithm for the machine cell formation problem. *International Journal of Production Economics*, 102, 1–21.

Grenouilleau, F., Legrain, A., Lahrichi, N., Rousseau, L.M. (2019). A set partitioning heuristic for the home health care routing problem. *European Journal of Operational Research*, 275, 295–303.

Grenouilleau, F., Lahrichi, N., Rousseau, L.M. (2020). New decomposition methods for home care scheduling with predefined visits. *Computers and Operations Research*, 115, 104–855.

Hewitt, M., Nowak, M., Nataraj, N. (2016). Planning strategies for home health care delivery. *Asia-Pacific Journal of Operational Research*, 33(5), 1650041.

Holland, J.H. (1975). *Adaptation in Natural and Artificial Systems: An Introductory Analysis with Applications to Biology, Control, and Artificial Intelligence*. University of Michigan Press, Ann Arbor, USA.

Issaoui, B., Zidi, I., Marcon, E., Ghedira, K. (2015). New multi-objective approach for the home care service problem based on scheduling algorithms and variable neighborhood descent. *Electronic Notes in Discrete Mathematics*, 47, 181–188.

Koeleman, P.M., Bhulai, S., Meersbergen, M. (2012). Optimal patient and personnel scheduling plocies for care-at-home service facilities. *European Journal of Operational Research*, 219(3), 557–563.

Lanzarone, E. and Matta, A. (2014). Robust nurse-to-patient assignment in home care services to minimize overtimes under continuity of care. *Operational Research for Health Care*, 3(2), 48–58.

Marcon, E., Chaabane, S., Sallez, Y., Bonte, T., Trentesaux, D. (2017). A multi-agent system based on reactive decision rules for solving the caregiver routing problem in HHC. *Simulation Modelling Practice Theory*, 74, 134–151.

Martinez, C., Espinousse, M-L., Di Mascolo, M. (2019). Re-planning in home healthcare: A review decomposition approach to minimize idle time for workers while ensuring continuity of care. *IFAC PapersOnLine*, 52(13), 654–659.

Mosquera, F., Smet, P., Berghe, G.V. (2019). Flexible home care scheduling. *Omega*, 83, 80–95.

Moussavi, S.E., Mahdjoub, M., Grunder, O. (2019). A metaheuristic approach to the integration of worker assignment and vehicle routing problems: Application to home health scheduling. *Expert Systems with Applications*, 125, 317–332.

Mutingi, M. and Mbohwa, C. (2012). A group genetic algorithm for the fleet size and mix vehicle routing problem. *IEEE Proceedings*, 1468–1472.

Mutingi, M. and Mbohwa, C. (2013). A home healthcare multi-agent system in a multi-objective environment. *SAIIE25 Proceedings*, 636, 1–8.

Nasir, J.A. and Kuo, Y.H. (2020). A decision support framework for home health care transportation with simultaneous multi-vehicle routing and staff scheduling synchronization. *Decision Support Systems*, 138, 113–361.

Nasir, J.A., Hussain, S., Dang, C. (2018). An integrated planning approach towards home health care, telehealth and patients group based care. *Journal of Network and Computer Applications*, 117, 30–41.

Nickel, S., Schröder, M., Steeg, J. (2012). Mid-term and short-term planning support for home health care services. *European Journal of Operational Research*, 219(3), 574–587.

Nikzad, E., Bashiri, M., Abbasi, B. (2020). A metaheuristic algorithm for stochastic home health care planning. *European Journal of Operational Research*, 288, 753–774.

Redjem, R., Kharraja, S., Marcon, E. (2011). Collaborative model for planning and scheduling caregivers' activities in homecare. *IFAC Proceedings Volumes*, 44, 2877–2882.

Shahnejat-Bushehri, S., Tavakkoli-Moghaddam, R., Momen, S., Ghasemkhani, A., Tavakkoli-Moghaddam, H. (2019). Home health care routing and scheduling problem considering temporal dependencies and perishability with simultaneous pickup and delivery. *IFAC PapersOnLine*, 52(13), 118–123.

Shi, Y., Boudouh, T., Grunder, O. (2017). A hybrid genetic algorithm for a home health care routing problem with time window and fuzzy demand. *Expert Systems with Applications*, 72, 160–176.

Shi, Y., Boudouh, T., Grunder, O. (2019). A robust optimization for a home health care routing and scheduling problem with consideration of uncertain travel service times. *Transportation Research Part E*, 128, 52–95.

Stojanova, A., Stojkovic, N., Kocaleva, M., Koceski, S. (2017). Agent-based solution of caregiver scheduling problem in home-care context. *14th International Conference on Informatics and Information Technologies*, Mavrovo, Macedonia, 7–9 April.

Vishnupriyan, S., Govindarajan, L., Prabhakaran, G., Ramachandran, K.P. (2008). Quality improvement in higher education through normalization of student feedback data using evolutionary algorithm. *Proceedings of International Journal of Applied Management and Technology*, 6(3).

Widmer, T. and Premm, M. (2015). Agent-based decision support for allocating caregiving resources in a dementia scenario. In *MATES 2015*, Müller, J.P., Ketter, W., Kaminka, G., Wagner, G., Bulling, N. (eds). Springer, Cham, Switzerland.

Wirnitzer, J., Heckmann, I., Meyer, A., Nickel, S. (2015). Patient-based nurse rostering in home care. *Operations Research for Health Care*, 8, 91–102

Xiao, L., Dridi, M., El Hassani, A.H. (2018). Mathematical model for the home health care scheduling and routing problem with flexible lunch break requirements. *IFAC PapersOnLine*, 51(11), 334–339.

Xie, Z. (2016). Decentralized and dynamic home health care resource scheduling using an agent-based model. PhD Thesis, Concordia University, Montreal, Canada.

Xie, Z.A. and Wang, C. (2017). A periodic repair algorithm for dynamic scheduling in home health care using agent-based model. *IEEE 21st International Conference on Computer Supported Cooperative Work in Design (CSCWD)*, 245–250, Wellington, New Zealand, 26–28 April.

3

Optimal Sizing of an Automated Dispensing Cabinet Under Adjacency Constraints

3.1. Introduction

The three main phases of the medication-use process are prescription, dispensing and administration. The prescription phase corresponds to writing and updating the prescription to the patient file. The dispensing phase corresponds to the validation of the prescription, its preparation and delivery of the drugs. The administration phase includes the preparation and administration of the drug to the patient. Different errors can occur throughout the three phases. In this study, we will focus on the errors that occur during the dispensing phase, with the aim of minimizing them. When properly utilized, automated dispensing cabinets can dramatically reduce medication selection errors in comparison to manual dispensing. However, errors can occur when filling the cabinet, and the improper placement of a product in the cabinet increases the likelihood that a patient will receive the wrong medication (Hyland *et al.* 2007). Therefore, decisions about how much medicine is stored and where it is located is critical to the reliability and safety of an automated cabinet.

To avoid dispensing errors, their causes should be eliminated. For example, confusion due to similarities in drug names between brand names (e.g. Sumial® and Luminal®) is a common cause of medication errors (Hoffman and Proulx 2003). Indeed, human factors, such as lack of attention, can lead to dispensing errors from poor selection of drugs with a similar sounding and/or similar name (similar

Chapter written by Khalid HACHEMI, Didier GOURC and François MARMIER.

sounding names or similar packaging). Some solutions and good practices are presented in Emmerton and Rizk (2012).

Several techniques exist to reduce administration errors. The use of capital letters in the writing of the names of drugs (López *et al.* 2011), as in Hydroxyzine and Hydralazine written HydrOXYzine, and HydrALAzine, can mark the difference. Another way to prevent administration errors is through the use of barcodes to identify drugs (Morriss *et al.* 2009; Poon *et al.* 2010; Hassink *et al.* 2012).

Several research studies have investigated the impact of the introduction of automated dispensing systems in pharmacies. In a study by Oswald and Caldwell (2007), the authors estimated the rate of filling and dispensing error before and after the implementation of an automated carousel system at the 613-bed Stanford University Hospital. They observed a drastic reduction in the error rate through the use of this system. In another study (Serrano *et al.* 2012), the authors analyzed the impact of the "Pyxis MedStation®" automated dispensing system in intensive care units (ICUs), both financially and in terms of human resources. By creating a medication list and using the "Sinfohspharmacy" management software, they showed that the monthly cost per patient with the Pyxis MedStation® system was reduced by 20.3%. The number of drugs in stock increased by 11.4%. In addition, less space was needed for storage and staff needed less time to perform distribution operations; on average, a reduction of two hours per day. Some researchers have studied the economic impact of the introduction of automated dispensing systems (Chapuis *et al.* 2015). Regarding automated dispensing cabinets, Pazour *et al.* (2012) addressed the problem of locating drugs inside the drawers of automated dispensing cabinets (ADC), in order to minimize human selection errors. They developed a quadratic optimization model, making it possible to determine the best storage locations, so as to avoid placing two similar drugs side by side, in order to reduce picking errors. However, solving full-size problems is not practical; the authors note that solving a twelve-drug, two-drawer problem using CPLEX10.1 fails to find an optimal solution due to memory limitations. Therefore, they proposed a heuristic solution approach. Hachemi and Alla (2013) addressed the problem of drug allocation in an ADC model cabinet using Petri nets. Their objective, seen from the perspective of a control problem, was to create a controller that prevented two incompatible drugs side by being placed side. The problem considered in this chapter is the prediction of the existence of a medication allocation solution based on the drawer dimensions of an ADC automated dispensing cabinet.

A 2011 American Society of Health-System Pharmacists (ASHP) investigation into the evaluation of practices and technologies related to drug dispensing and administration, involving 1,401 hospitals in the United States, found that the adoption of new technologies is changing the philosophy of drug distribution and health information. Indeed, health information, including patient drug profiles, is increasingly electronic, allowing easier access to patient information by all nurses and pharmacists. In addition, drug distribution is increasingly decentralized, and medication is being kept closer to patients (Pedersen *et al.* 2012). This study noted that 89% of hospitals used automated dispensing cabinets.

This same survey was conducted again in 2014 and found that 97% of the hospitals surveyed used automated dispensing cabinets (ADCs) (Pedersen *et al.* 2015), confirming the trend towards decentralized drug delivery systems, which have the advantage of reducing costs and minimizing delays by bringing medication closer to the point of care.

A recent study further highlighted the role of ADCs in reducing dispensing errors (Fanning *et al.* 2016) by ensuring the physical separation of similar drugs and the incorporation of LED warning lights to help guide the operator to the correct compartment.

In this chapter, we discuss the problem of determining the feasibility of allocating drugs in an automated dispensing cabinet (ADC). The problem is to determine the boundary conditions necessary for the allocation of drugs to the different compartments of a cabinet, knowing that there are drugs that should not be placed in neighboring compartments due to the risk of confusion, which could lead to distribution errors. In this chapter, we infer by "incompatible medication" to drugs with either a very similar appearance, nomenclature, packaging, dosage, frequency of application, level of risk and/or strength of dosage, as mentioned in Pazour and Meller (2012).

To achieve this, the chapter is broken down into multiple sections. An introduction is given in section 3.1. In section 3.2, we present the automated dispensing cabinet and the resulting allocation problem. In section 3.3, we develop an algebraic model for the computation of boundary conditions and the formulation of the maximum permissive target problem (MPTP). A full-size numerical application is given in section 3.4. Finally, we present the conclusions and future areas for study in section 3.5.

3.2. Problem statement

In this section, we give the description of the automated dispensing cabinet (ADC) and the drug allocation problem, as well as the notation and definitions used in the mathematical formulation.

3.2.1. *Description of the assignment problem*

The problem is to assign the different existing drugs to the compartments of each drawer, with the knowledge that there are drugs that should not be placed in neighboring compartments (sharing one side), due to the risk of confusion, which may lead to dispensing errors. The confusion arises from the similarity that can exist between two drugs. Therefore, a list of similar drugs is given by an incompatibility matrix (the pairing of drugs) whose elements are equal to 1 or 0, with the respective values indicating whether the two drugs are incompatible or not. Note that we generate a binary matrix from the similarity matrix, introduced in Pazour *et al.* (2012), by applying a binarization of the similarity matrix with an adaptive threshold. We propose to study the feasibility of the allocation problem (by not placing incompatible drugs in adjacent compartments). In order to do this, we try to determine the properties (boundary conditions) that the incompatibility matrix must satisfy in order to guarantee the existence of an acceptable solution.

3.2.2. *Notations and definitions*

p: number of compartments per column, $p \in N^* - \{1\}$ (see Figure 3.1), where N^* is the set of positive integers.

q: number of compartments per row, $q \in N^* - \{1\}$ (see Figure 3.1); drawers must have at least two rows and two columns to avoid having compartments with a single adjacent compartment (singular case).

n: number of drawers.

m: number of compartments in a drawer (drawer capacity); $m = p \times q$.

d: number of medications to be assigned to the drawer, $d \in N^*$.

S: similarity matrix of incompatible medications of dimension $d \times d$, such that $S_{jk} \in [0,1]$, where a value of 0 indicates the lowest degree of incompatibility between two drugs, while a value of 1 represents the highest degree of incompatibility between two drugs. We suppose that $S_{jj} = 0$.

I: binary matrix of S of dimension $d \times d$.

$$I_{jk} = \begin{cases} 1 \; if \; drugs \; j \; and \; k \; are \; incompatible \; (if \; S_{jk} \geq y) \\ 0 \;\; else \end{cases}$$

with j, k: medication indices to allocate the drawer, $(j, k) \in [1, d]$.

y: binarization threshold, $y \in]0,1]$.

Note that the matrix I is symmetric, that is, $I_{kr} = I_{rk}$. In the following, we will denote by the matrix I the incompatibility matrix. From matrix I, we can deduce the number of incompatible drug pairs b as follows:

$$\boldsymbol{b} = \sum_{j=1}^{j=d} \sum_{k=j}^{k=d} I_{jk} \qquad [3.1]$$

r: vector of dimension $1xd$ representing the number of occurrences of each drug in the set of incompatible drug pairs, $r \in N$, it can be deduced from matrix I as follows:

$$r_j = \sum_{k=1}^{d} I_{jk} \quad \forall j \in [1, d] \qquad [3.2]$$

r': vector of dimension 1×3 of the maximum (tolerated) appearances of a drug in the set of incompatible pairs. Dimension 3 comes from the number of types of compartments (see Definition 3.1 below).

w: vector of dimension 1×3 representing the number of compartments of each type.

e: the maximum (tolerated) number of incompatible drug pairs that can be placed in a drawer.

v: the number of combinations between every two adjacent compartments of the drawer.

DEFINITION 3.1.– The type of compartment depends on the number of adjacent compartments (sharing a side) that a particular compartment has. Therefore, a compartment, depending on its position in the drawer, has 2 (type 1), 3 (type 2) or 4 (type 3) adjacent compartments (see Figure 3.2).

DEFINITION 3.2.– We define the vector $c = [2 \quad 3 \quad 4]^T$. It represents the number of shared sides for each type of compartment.

Thus, a vector $w = [4 \quad 8 \quad 4]$ means that in the considered drawer, the number of type 1 compartments is 4, type 2 is 8 and type 3 is 4.

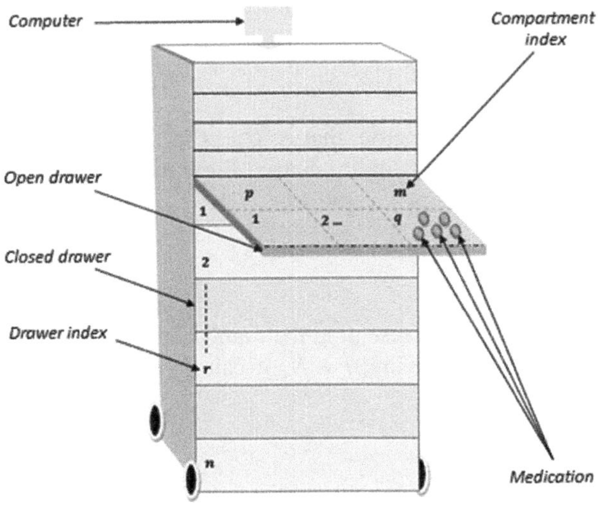

Figure 3.1. *Drawer configuration*

Type 1	*Type 2*	*Type 1*
Type 2	*Type 3*	*Type 2*
Type 1	*Type 2*	*Type 1*

Figure 3.2. *Types of compartments in a* 3×3 *drawer*

3.3. Mathematical formulation

In order to formulate the problem, we consider several dimensions of the drawer, and each and every time, we calculate the maximum number of drug appearances the drawer can tolerate, that is, allowing for an assignment that avoids placing incompatible medications side by side. In addition, we will take the case where $d = m$.

3.3.1. *Determination of boundary conditions*

The boundary conditions of the assignment problem will be determined from the incompatibility matrix I containing the maximum number of incompatible drug pairs that allows for an acceptable solution. Here, we denote this matrix through the maximum-permissive matrix.

Special case: a square drawer where $p = q$. We can determine the maximum possible number of incompatible pairs by calculating the number of combinations of two elements among d; thus, we have:

$$C_d^2 = \frac{d!}{2!\,(d-2)!} = \frac{(d-1)\times d}{2} \qquad [3.\ 3]$$

Note that the maximum number (upper limit) of incompatible drug pairs **that can be placed in a drawer** is given by equation [3.4].

$$e = C_d^2 - v \qquad [3.4]$$

Such that: $v = \frac{1}{2}(4 \times 2 + 2(q-2) \times 3 + 2(p-2) \times 3 + (p-2)(q-2) \times 4)$

$$v = 4 + 3(p + q - 4) + 2(p-2)(q-2) \qquad [3.5]$$

The vector r' showing the number of maximum (tolerated) appearances of a drug in the set of incompatible pairs can be determined from equation [3.6].

This expression comes from the fact that each occurrence of incompatible drug pairs corresponds to 1 shared side.

$$r' = (p \times q).Id - c - Id$$

By replacing $p.q$ by d, we find:

$$r' = d \times Id - c - Id, such\ that\!: Id = \begin{bmatrix}1\\1\\1\end{bmatrix} \qquad [3.6]$$

By observing the evolution of the vector w as a function of the size of the drawer, we can easily deduce its expression according to the following formula:

$$w = [4 \quad (p-2) \times 4 \quad (p-2)^2] \qquad [3.7]$$

The boundary conditions are given by the vectors r' and w as follows:

r' gives the maximum size (maximum number of drugs) of the set of drugs assigned to three types of drugs.

w gives the maximum number of occurrences for each type of drug.

In general, for a square drawer: in order to have a possible assignment, it is necessary that:

The number of medications with $r'[1]$ (type 1) appearances <u>should be $\leq w[1]$</u> [3.8]

The number of medications with $r'[2]$ (type 2) appearances <u>should be</u> $\leq w[2]$ [3.9]

The number of medications with $r'[3]$ (type 3) appearances <u>should be</u> $\leq w[3]$ [3.10]

with $w\,[1] + w\,[2] + w\,[3] = d$

It should be mentioned that these are necessary but not sufficient conditions. This means that, if the conditions are not met, it is necessarily deduced that there is no possible assignment. Otherwise, we cannot deduce the existence, or not, of a possible solution.

General case: all drawers with $p \neq q$. We can generalize the previous results (conditions [3.8], [3.9] and [3.10]) for any drawer as follows:

$$w = [4 \quad 2(p-2) + 2(q-2) \quad (p-2)(q-2)]$$

$$w = [4 \quad 2(p+q-4) \quad (p-2)(q-2)] \qquad [3.11]$$

Expressions [3.4], [3.5] and [3.6] remain applicable to the general case.

3.3.2. *Problem solving approach*

We will develop a method of resolution based on the previous boundary conditions, in order to determine if an assignment solution exists or not. Before presenting the results, let us first give some definitions.

DEFINITION 3.3.– Let I be an incompatibility matrix. A binary matrix I' of the same dimension as I is defined as a matrix complementary to the matrix I, such that:

$$I'_{jk} = \begin{cases} 0 \ \ if \ \ (I_{jk} = 1) \ or \ (j = k) \\ \leq 1 \ else \end{cases}$$

DEFINITION 3.4.– A matrix I is defined as a maximum permissive matrix if it strictly respects the upper limits of w in the boundary conditions, that is:

The number of medications with $r'[1]$ (type 1) appearances <u>should be</u> $= w[1]$

The number of medications with $r'[2]$ (type 2) appearances <u>should be</u> $= w[2]$

The number of medications with $r'[3]$ (type 3) appearances <u>should be</u> $= w[3]$

with $w\,[1] + w\,[2] + w\,[3] = d$

The basic idea consists of transforming the given matrix I into a maximum permissive matrix by transforming certain 0s in the initial matrix into 1. Thus, we can state the following theorem.

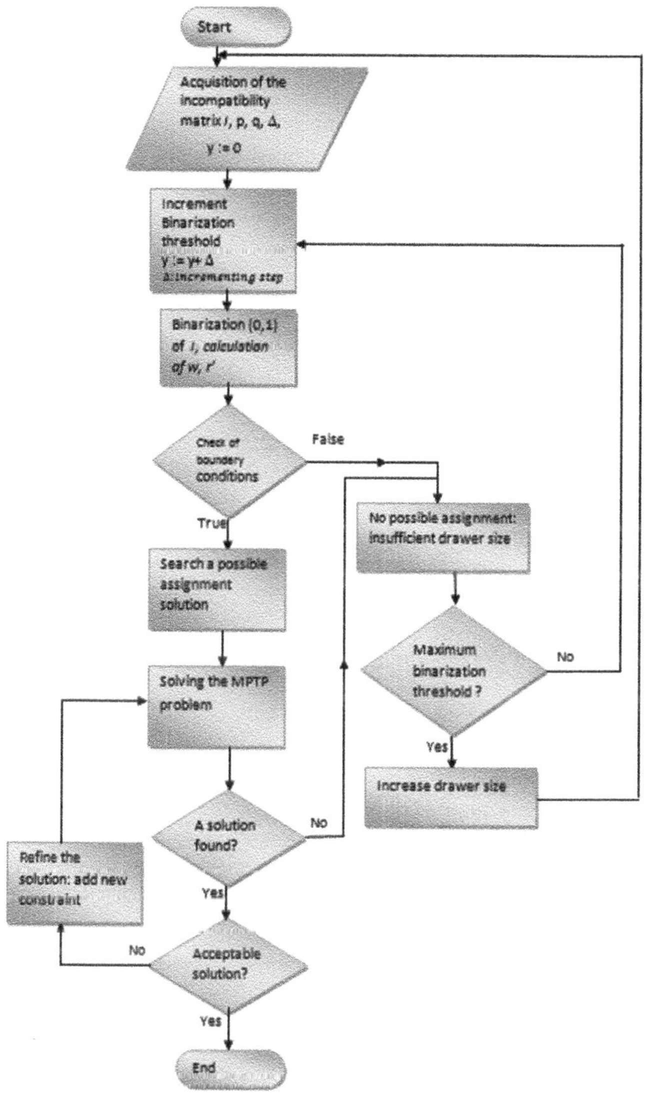

Figure 3.3. *Flowchart of the allocation problem decision process*

THEOREM 3.1.– Given an incompatibility matrix I, if there is no complementary matrix I' such that: $I + I' = R$, where R is maximum permissive, then an acceptable solution for the assignment problem does not exist. Indeed:

$$(For\ I\ \nexists\ I' : I + I' = R) \rightarrow \nexists\ solution$$

PROOF OF THEOREM 3.1.– We use a proof by contradiction. Suppose that the proposition given in the theorem is false, that is, its inverse is true: $for\ I\ \forall\ I'(complementary\ matrix\ of\ I)$:

$I + I' \neq R$, where R is the maximum permissive and an acceptable solution exists. However, when the solution exists, it must respect $I + I' = R$ (in contradiction with the assumption). Therefore, the assumption is false and the proposition of Theorem 3.1 is true.

On the basis of Theorem 3.1, we construct a mixed integer linear program (MILP) model whose goal is to find a complementary matrix I' such that: $I + I' = R$, where R is the maximum permissive. In this chapter, we refer to this problem as the *maximum permissive target problem* (MPTP). Hence, we develop an algorithm capable of predicting the non-existence of an acceptable assignment according to an incompatibility matrix I. This makes it possible to provide decision support for the resizing of drawers or the relaxation of incompatibility constraints by incrementing the binarization threshold. Figure 3.3 shows the flowchart of the decision process using a drawer allocation resolution algorithm.

Decision variables:

I': binary matrix S of dimension $d * d$ such that:

$$I'_{jk} = \begin{cases} 0\ if\ \ (I_{jk} = 1)\ or\ (j = k) \\ \qquad\quad \leq 1\ \ else \end{cases} \qquad [3.12]$$

Note that I' is a binary matrix, that is:

$$I'_{jk} \in \{0,1\}\ \forall\ j \in [1,d],\ \ \forall k \in [1,d] \qquad [3.13]$$

Recall that I is also a binary matrix, that is:

$$I_{jk} \in \{0,1\}\ \forall\ j \in [1,d],\ \ \forall k \in [1,d] \qquad [3.14]$$

Model:

$$\boldsymbol{min} \sum_{j=1}^{d} \sum_{k=1}^{d} I_{jk} + I'_{jk} \qquad [3.15]$$

$$s.c. \quad \sum_{k=1}^{d} I_{jk} + I'_{jk} \leq r'_s \quad \forall j \in [1,d] \qquad [3.16]$$

$$\sum_{k=1}^{d} I_{jk} + I'_{jk} \geq r'_l \quad \forall j \in [1,d] \qquad [3.17]$$

$$I'_{jk} = 0 \;\; if\; ((I_{jk} = 1) or (j = k)) \;\; \forall j \in [1,d], \;\; \forall k \in [1,d] \qquad [3.18]$$

$$I'_{jk} \leq 1 \;\; if\; I_{jk} = 0 \;\; \forall j \in [1,d], \;\; \forall k \in [1,d] \qquad [3.19]$$

$$\sum_{j=1}^{d} \sum_{k=1}^{d} I_{jk} + I'_{jk} = \sum_{i=1}^{3} r'_i \, w_i \qquad [3.20]$$

$$I'_{jk} \in \{0,1\} \; \forall j \in [1,d], \;\; \forall k \in [1,d] \qquad [3.21]$$

The objective [3.15] minimizes the number of 1s in the matrix I', that is, it minimizes the number of pairs of incompatible medications added to obtain a maximum permissive matrix $(I + I')$. The constraint [3.16] ensures that the number of incompatible medications for each drug does not exceed the upper limit stated by the vector r'. The constraint [3.17] ensures that the number of incompatible pairs for each medication is greater than or equal to the lower limit stated by the vector r'. The constraints [3.18] and [3.19] ensure that the matrix I' is complementary to I. The constraint [3.20] allows for the addition of the appropriate number of 1 (number of incompatible pairs) to the matrix I', according to the limits set out by the boundary conditions. Finally, the elements of I'_{jk} are forced to be binary in [3.21].

3.4. Application example

In this example we consider an industrial size problem with a 6X5 drawer, that is, $p = 5$, $q = 6$. Therefore, the number of drugs to be assigned is: $d = p.q = 30$. The incompatibility matrix I after binarization with a threshold of 0.25 is given in Table 3.1. Since the matrix is symmetrical, we only present the upper half.

The boundary conditions of a 6X5 drawer are given as follows: The number of medications with 27 (type 1) appearances should be ≤ 4. The number of medications with 26 (type 2) appearances should be ≤ 14. The number of medications with 25 (type 3) appearances should be ≤ 12.

In this example, we can see that the boundary conditions are met: the number of drugs with 27 occurrences (type 1) is equal to 4, the number of drugs with 26 occurrences (type 2) is equal to 6 and the number of drugs with 25 occurrences (type 3) is equal to 8. Although the boundary conditions are met, the MILP does not provide any solution to the MPTP. We thus conclude that the size of the drawer is insufficient to place all of the drugs without placing incompatible medications in adjacent compartments. This requires increasing either the binarization threshold or the size of the drawer, in order to provide a possible assignment. As such, we have to choose the second option if we do not want to lose too much information from the incompatibility matrix I.

I_{jk}	1	2	3	4	5	6	7	8	9	10	11	12	13	14	15	16	17	18	19	20	21	22	23	24	25	26	27	28	29	30	r_j
1	0	1	1	1	1	1	1	1	1	1	1	1	1	1	1	1	1	1	1	1	1	1	1	1	1	1	1	1	0	0	27
2		0	1	1	1	1	1	1	1	1	1	1	1	1	1	1	1	1	1	1	1	1	1	1	1	1	1	0	0	0	26
3			0	1	1	1	1	1	1	1	1	1	1	1	1	1	1	1	1	1	1	1	1	1	1	1	0	0	0	0	25
4				0	1	1	1	1	1	1	1	1	1	1	1	1	1	1	1	1	1	1	1	1	1	1	1	1	0	0	27
5					0	1	1	1	1	1	1	1	1	1	1	1	1	1	1	1	1	1	1	1	1	1	1	1	0	0	27
6						0	1	1	1	1	1	1	1	1	1	1	1	1	1	1	1	1	1	1	1	1	1	1	0	0	27
7							0	1	1	1	1	1	1	1	1	1	1	1	1	1	1	1	1	1	1	1	1	0	0	0	26
8								0	1	1	1	1	1	1	1	1	1	1	1	1	1	1	1	1	1	1	1	0	0	0	22
9									0	1	1	1	1	1	1	1	1	1	1	1	1	1	1	1	1	1	1	0	0	0	26
10										0	1	1	1	1	1	1	1	1	1	1	1	1	1	1	1	0	0	0	0	0	24
11											0	1	1	1	1	1	1	0	1	1	1	0	1	1	1	1	1	0	0	0	24
12												0	1	1	1	1	1	1	1	1	1	1	1	0	1	0	1	0	0	0	24
13													0	1	1	1	1	1	1	0	1	1	1	1	1	1	1	0	0	0	25
14														0	1	1	1	1	0	1	0	1	1	1	1	1	1	0	0	0	24
15															0	1	1	1	1	1	1	1	1	1	1	1	1	0	0	0	26
16																0	1	1	1	1	1	1	1	1	1	1	1	0	0	0	26
17																	0	1	1	1	1	1	1	1	1	1	1	0	0	0	26
18																		0	1	1	1	1	1	1	1	1	1	0	0	0	25
19																			0	1	1	1	0	1	1	1	1	0	0	0	24
20																				0	1	1	1	1	1	1	1	0	0	0	25
21																					0	1	1	1	1	1	1	0	0	0	25
22																						0	1	1	1	1	1	0	0	0	25
23																							0	1	0	1	1	0	0	0	24
24																								0	1	1	1	0	0	0	25
25																									0	1	1	0	0	0	25
26																										0	1	0	0	0	24
27																											0	0	0	0	24
28																												0	0	0	4
29																													0	0	0
30																														0	0

Table 3.1. *Incompatibility matrix I after binarization (y = 0.25)*

Finally, let us note that sometimes the solution found by the solver does not yield an acceptable solution. We thus propose a second supervision step which will check the matrix (I + I'), according to the inter-incompatibilities between the types of drugs as follows: for each drawer size, it is easy to determine the 3 × 3 matrix for which the items represent the maximum number of incompatibilities between one type of medication and another. Let Z be this matrix.

Z_{kj}: is the maximum (tolerated) number of incompatibilities of each medication of type j with a k-type medication. For example, for a 3 × 3 drawer, Z is equal to:

$$Z = \begin{bmatrix} 3 & 2 & 1 \\ 2 & 3 & 0 \\ 4 & 0 & 0 \end{bmatrix} \quad [3.22]$$

We can find another solution by adding the constraint, representing the previous solution, to the MILP of the MPTP. The same procedure is repeated until an acceptable solution respecting the limits of the matrix Z is found.

3.5. Conclusion

In this chapter, we have discussed the problem of determining the feasibility of assigning medication to an automated dispensing cabinet, based on the size of the drawer and the number of incompatible medication pairs. We have developed an algebraic model to determine the boundary conditions for the maximum number of medication occurrences for all incompatible medication pairs. This number determines the upper limit of occurrence, which should not be exceeded; otherwise, there is no acceptable solution to the problem, that is, drug distribution, ensuring that incompatible drug pairs are not placed side by side. The results of this study, to our knowledge, constitute an original contribution to the optimal resolution of the assignment problem of an ADC. Indeed, the resolution of the proposed assignment problem is more efficient with a faster computation time than the quadratic assignment problem approached in Pazour and Meller (2012). This is due to an elegant solving method that efficiently exploits boundary conditions, so as to identify a possible solution to the MPTP using an MILP. The use of the developed approach makes it possible to study whether a feasible allocation of the medications inside the drawer is possible. If the assignment is not feasible, it is recommended that the size of the drawer, be increased, instead of increasing the binarization threshold, which will incur information losses on the incompatibility matrix. Future studies should explore the balanced choice between a reasonable binarization threshold and an increase in the size of the drawer, according to the preferences of the decision maker, with an optimized compromise between safety and economy. To this end, it would be very interesting to develop an indicator capable of measuring the quality of a solution, in order to provide useful information for the decision-maker.

3.6. References

Chapuis, C., Bedouch, P., Detavernier, M., Durand, M., Francony, G., Lavagne, P., Payen, J.F. (2015). Automated drug dispensing systems in the intensive care unit: A financial analysis. *Critical Care*, 19(1), 318.

Emmerton, L.M. and Rizk, M.F. (2012). Look-alike and sound-alike medicines: Risks and "solutions". *International Journal of Clinical Pharmacy*, 34(1), 4–8.

Fanning, L., Jones, N., Manias, E. (2016). Impact of automated dispensing cabinets on medication selection and preparation error rates in an emergency department: A prospective and direct observational before-and-after study. *Journal of Evaluation in Clinical Practice*, 22(2), 156–163.

Hachemi, K. and Alla, H. (2013). Assignment of drugs in an automated drug dispensing cabinet: An approach based on petri-net controller synthesis. *8th International Conference on Integrated Design and Production (CPI2013)*, Tlemcen, Algeria, 21–23 October.

Hassink, J.J.M., Jansen, M.M.P.M., Helmons, P.J. (2012). Effects of bar code-assisted medication administration (BCMA) on frequency, type and severity of medication administration errors: A review of the literature. *European Journal of Hospital Pharmacy: Science and Practice*, 19(5), 489–494.

Hoffman, J.M. and Proulx, S.M. (2003). Medication errors caused by confusion of drug names. *Drug Safety*, 26(7), 445–452.

Hyland, S., Koczmara, C., Salsman, B., Musing, E.L.S., Greenall, J. (2007). Optimizing the use of automated dispensing cabinets. *The Canadian Journal of Hospital Pharmacy*, 60(5), 332–334.

López, M.J.O., Muñoz, R.M., Barba, M.S., Sazatornil, R.A., Crespo, A.A., Jiménez, M.A., Vicedo, T.B., Ordoñana, G.C., TML Working Group (2011). Development of a list of look-alike drug names with recommended tall man letters. *FarmaciaHospitalaria* (English Edition), 35(5), 225–235.

Morriss, Jr., F.H., Abramowitz, P.W., Nelson, S.P., Milavetz, G., Michael, S.L., Gordon, S.N., Cook, E.F. (2009). Effectiveness of a barcode medication administration system in reducing preventable adverse drug events in a neonatal intensive care unit: A prospective cohort study. *The Journal of Pediatrics*, 154(3), 363–368.

Oswald, S. and Caldwell, R. (2007). Dispensing error rate after implementation of an automated pharmacy carousel system. *American Journal of Health-System Pharmacy*, 64(13), 1427–1431.

Pazour, J.A. and Meller, R.D. (2012). A multiple-drawer medication layout problem in automated dispensing cabinets. *Health Care Management Science*, 15(4), 339–354.

Pedersen, C.A., Schneider, P.J., Scheckelhoff, D.J. (2012). ASHP national survey of pharmacy practice in hospital settings: Dispensing and administration 2011. *American Journal of Health-System Pharmacy*, 69(9), 768–785.

Pedersen, C.A., Schneider, P.J., Scheckelhoff, D.J. (2015). ASHP national survey of pharmacy practice in hospital settings: Dispensing and administration 2014. *American Journal of Health-System Pharmacy*, 72(13), 1119–1137.

Poon, E.G., Keohane, C.A., Yoon, C.S., Ditmore, M., Bane, A., Levtzion-Korach, O., Churchill, W.W. (2010). Effect of bar-code technology on the safety of medication administration. *New England Journal of Medicine*, 362(18), 1698–1707.

Serrano, P.S., Pin, A.C., Copa, P.C., Rodriguez, N.P. (2012). Introduction of an automated drug dispensing system in an intensive care unit. *European Journal of Hospital Pharmacy: Science and Practice*, 19(2), 141–141.

4

Validation of an Automated and Targeted Pharmaceutical Analysis Tool at the CHU de Liège

4.1. Introduction

Medication flow in a hospital is a complex and multidisciplinary process (Mahé 2014). It includes clinical pathways (prescription, distribution, administration) and logistics (supply, transport, storage). In addition to the adverse drugs events, medication errors are a major problem for patient safety. They are defined by the Belgian national agency of drug safety and health products (*Agence nationale de sécurité du medicament et des produits de santé*, ANSM) as "the omission or unintentional performance of an act occurring during a care process involving a medicine, which may be the source of a risk or an adverse event for the patient" (Durand 2012). Medication errors are frequent, costly and have an impact on clinical practice. Several studies have analyzed the occurrence of medication errors within the various stages of the medication flow. One of these studies was conducted by a French health product safety agency (*Agence française de sécurité sanitaire des produits de santé*, often abbreviated to AFSSAPS) (AFSSAPS 2009). According to this study, medication errors were mainly related to administration (57%) and distribution (15%) errors. However, other studies report prescribing errors of up to 56% (Mahé 2014).

Securing each step in the hospital medication flow constitutes a major challenge. Computerization can be a key element of daily security, in particular, by linking the

---

Chapter written by Sophie STREEL, Nathalie MAES, Véronique GONCETTE, Laurence SEIDEL, Denis MENAGER, Adelin ALBERT, Philippe KOLH and Didier MAESEN.

electronic prescription service (EPS) to a clinical decision support system (CDSS) (Figure 4.1).

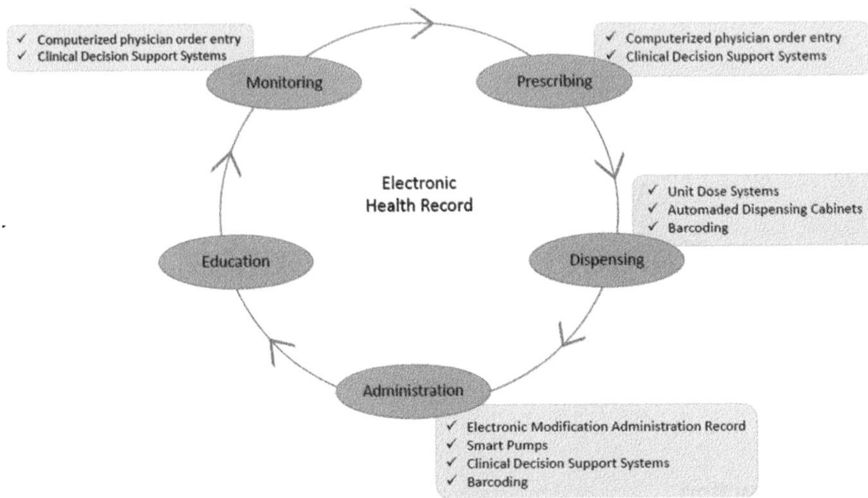

Figure 4.1. *Presentation of IT solutions throughout the medication process (Seidling and Bates 2016)*

The *CHU de Liège* is a large university teaching facility with a capacity of 1,015 beds and four distinct sites. There are about 3,400 outpatient visits every day, 250 emergency admissions and 160 new hospitalizations. The CHU de Liège employs more than 900 physicians working in 50 clinical departments, covering all medical disciplines. Based on an average of nine medications per patient, the total number of drug prescriptions is estimated at 6,480 per day.

The hospital information system (HIS) at the CHU de Liège has reached Level 6 on the HIMSS EMRAM scale (out of 7 Levels), which can be viewed as quite a technological achievement. Currently, a little more than 80% of the beds benefit from the electronic prescription service (EPS) and the medication administration plan, coupled with a basic CDSS, which works on the basis of a comparison with the available databases (drug interactions, duplicates) and sends alerts to the HIS for prescribing physicians. The pharmacy uses robots which are controlled by the EPS and the medication stock management system. The robots, which identify each medication individually, are connected to the EPS and associate patient an identifier, dosage, route and time for administration with each patient. Automated dispensation cabinets are also connected to the prescription medication information

(PMI) and only deliver prescribed medications. Medication administration security is deployed in the care units via a barcode applied to all drugs and validated via PDAs (Personal Digital Assistant).

In 2014, the CHU de Liège decided to enter into an accreditation process to warrant optimal risk and safety management and establish the reputation of the hospital. The benchmark chosen was that of the Joint Commission International (JCI 2017), selected for the quality of its standards and the consideration of university status. Its chapter on "medication management and use (MMU)" recommends that good medication management should be associated with a double review of each prescription: checking the suitability of the medication in relation to the patient and their clinical needs when prescribing medication checking and the suitability of the medication prescribed during administration.

The hospital pharmacy carries out a partially targeted verification of treatments, but not in a systematic and exhaustive way. It includes an analysis of dosages, allergies, duplicates, demographics, physiological and biological constants of the patient. However, systematic validation is not possible as it would consume too much in terms of the staffing resources.

The objective of this study was to establish and validate a targeted computerized pharmaceutical analysis tool compliant with the institutional criteria of quality and external accreditation. It also aimed to assess the acceptance rate of interventions by the hospital pharmacist that differ from those of the prescribing physician.

4.2. Methods

The implementation of the pharmaceutical tool began in 2018 with the creation of working groups, consisting of experts in each field, defining the different classes of high-risk drugs and the declarations of serious adverse events within the institution. These groups were set up to formulate risk reduction strategies for one or more stages of the medication circuit. These recommendations made it possible to prioritize the algorithms to be developed.

Presented in the form of decision trees, the pharmaceutical validation algorithms detail each recommendation step by step, going from the most general to the most specific information.

At the same time, the IT tool was developed internally by IT specialists from hand drawn diagrams.

The validation of the tool was done in 2019 by comparing a sample of prescriptions over a period of 21 days. Comparisons were made between:

– each unsuitably qualified prescription identified by the computerized tool was checked by a pharmacist (reference);

– each suitable or unsuitable prescription by a referent pharmacist who had the algorithms in paper format (control).

The sample of prescriptions was drawn from prescriptions to patients hospitalized during the period under consideration and belonging to a department that uses PMI; only patients with a situation listed in the four algorithms were included (Figure 4.2).

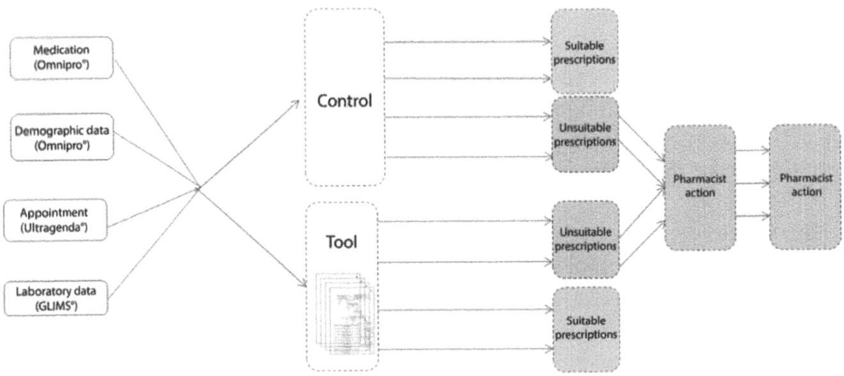

Figure 4.2. *Schematic representation of the study. For a color version of this figure, see www.iste.co.uk/chaabane/healthcare.zip*

The comparison was carried out using a 2 x 2 contingency table cross-classifying the decisions made by the computerized tool and the referring pharmacist (without the tool) considered as the "gold standard". The sensitivity and specificity of the algorithms were calculated; sensitivity was set to at least 95% for an algorithm to be validated. Discrepancies between manual and electronic decisions were analyzed in detail.

The tool acceptance rate was measured on the basis of the same sample of prescriptions by calculating the ratio between the number of procedures performed by prescribing physicians and the number of procedures that were followed. The reasons for not following the procedures were analyzed in detail.

4.3. Results

4.3.1. *Creation of algorithms*

The writing of the algorithms differed depending on the objective sought. This involved detecting either the absence of treatment (the algorithm searches for a pathological situation described in the patient files) or inadequate treatment (the algorithm searches for a drug based on its ATC code).

Four specific themes were selected, and the corresponding algorithms were created:

– detect the unsuitable prescriptions of anticoagulants;

– detect the absence of immunosuppressive management or inadequate management of immunosuppression;

– detect contraindications in renal failure;

– detect the use of contraindicated medications during pregnancy.

Each algorithm was validated institutionally by the corresponding working group via questionnaires.

4.3.2. *IT tool development*

The data necessary for the decision trees were extracted from the HIS: medical records, laboratory data, appointment scheduling, etc. Medicines were identified according to their full ATC code, to extend the scope of action of the IT tool beyond the specialties present in the hospital therapeutic formulary (personal medications, substitution in the event of company breakups, etc.).

From the data, the IT tool identified and qualified the prescription as unsuitable (alert) or suitable (no alert). The list of prescriptions was subject to a report (web-report) containing the patient references, date and time, type (name of the algorithm) and alert (Yes/No), as well as a description of the information used for automatic validation (Figure 4.4). The hospital pharmacist then noted down her remark on the alert and, if necessary, intervened with the prescribing physician. A pharmaceutical analysis dashboard was made available, allowing prescriptions to be “filtered” by *Day*, *Site*, *Type*, *Level* and according to whether they had been *Handled* or not.

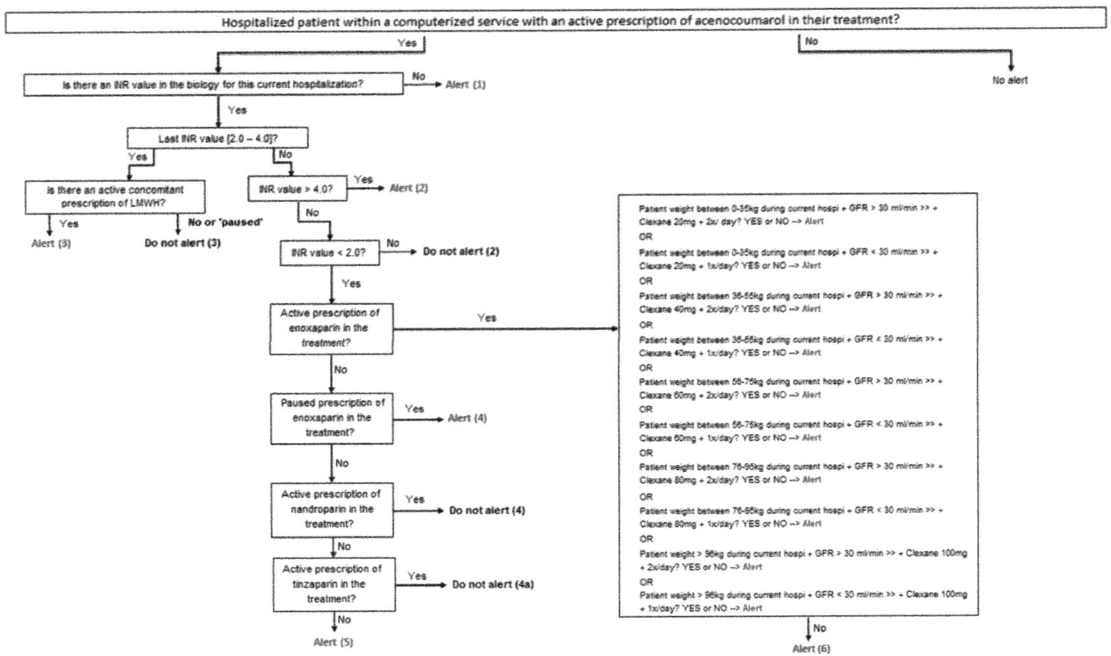

Figure 4.3. *Example of a decision tree developed and institutionally validated*

BY-1A Médecine A

Patients	Type	Level	Message
	IMMUNOSUPPRESSION	Do not alert	Presence of transplant for the patient. Drug prescription found: Tarcolimus. Mycophenolicacid. Blood dosage (9.2) in bio found.
	SINTROM	Do not alert	Prescription for acenocoumarol: INR less than 2 (=1.11) and prescription for enoxaparin found CLEXANE 60 MG 0.6 ML S and Dosage(s): 1 amp. ser. 2 x a day. CLEXANE 60 MG 0.6 ML S CLEXANE 80 MG 0.8 ML S and Dosage(s): 1 amp. ser. 2 x a day. GFR value found > 60 (04/08/2019 10:27:00) Weight = 75kg

Figure 4.4. *Translated extract from the "web-report" generated by the automated pharmaceutical analysis tool*

The electronic (algorithmic) tool was first beta-tested. This step consisted of verifying the accuracy of the result of the IT integration against the requirements or situations described in the algorithms. Computer adaptations were made until a perfect agreement was obtained between electronically derived results and the manual application of the decision tree by the hospital pharmacist using the HIS.

4.3.3. *Tool validation*

A total of 857 prescriptions obtained during the 21-day study period were validated separately by two pharmacists (the control with the tool and the referent without the tool).

Of these prescriptions, 419 (48.9%) were for the "Sintrom" algorithm, 329 (38.4%) were for "immunosuppression", 69 (8.1%) were for "contraindications of renal failure" and 40 (4.7%) were for "pregnancy".

Table 4.1 gives the comparison of pharmaceutical validations with or without the tool. With the pharmaceutical validation tool, 339 (40%) prescriptions generated an alert. The sensitivity of the IT tool, that is the probability that the tool will detect unsuitable prescriptions specified by the gold standard, was equal to 98% (196/201). The specificity, or namely the probability that the tool will correctly define a prescription as suitable, was 78% (513/656). In addition, the positive predictive value (PPV), namely the probability that a prescription detected as unsuitable by the algorithm is actually unsuitable, was 58% (196/339). Likewise, the negative predictive value (NPV), that is the probability that a prescription detected as suitable by the algorithm is actually suitable, was equal to 99% (513/518).

		Alert without the pharmaceutical validation tool (reference)		
		No (suitable)	Yes (unsuitable)	Total
Alert with the pharmaceutical validation tool (control)	No (suitable)	513	5	518
	Yes (unsuitable)	143	196	339
	Total	656	201	857

Table 4.1. *Comparison of pharmaceutical validations with or without the computerized tool (N = 857 prescription lines)*

The decision capabilities differed slightly between the four algorithms, with 100% sensitivity for "contraindications for renal failure" and 70% specificity for the algorithm "immunosuppression".

The identification of the five "false-negative" prescriptions considered suitable by the tool but actually unsuitable by the gold standard led to an adaptation of the algorithms. A total of 143 "false-positive" prescriptions (unsuitable by the tool but suitable by the referent) were also analyzed in detail. The majority (N = 61) was related to the quality of the extracted data needed by the computerized tool decision trees (erroneous, inconsistent or insufficiently specified data in the HIS, non-encoded processing). For 31 other cases, supplementary data arrived after computer extraction. In fact, two data extraction periods were programmed per day, at times when the HIS was less used, in order to avoid slowing down the operations.

Based on the sample of 857 prescriptions corresponding to 1 of the 4 algorithms in place, there were 74 interventions made by the pharmacist to the prescribing physician based on the pharmaceutical tool. Of the recommendations made during these interventions, 60 were followed, yielding an acceptance rate of 81%.

Interventions were carried out using messages in the HIS addressed directly to the prescribing physician; only interventions considered urgent by the pharmacist were done by direct telephone contact. Non-followed-up interventions were explained by, for example, the absence of the prescribing physician (e.g. a day after being on call). In the other cases, the HIS data available to the pharmacist were either partial or erroneous.

4.4. Discussion and conclusion

The study made it possible to set up an automatic pharmaceutical validation tool. Moreover, the tool was assessed statistically in terms of decision ability (sensitivity and specificity), giving more credit to the procedure used. Overall, sensitivity was high (98%) whence avoiding risky situations going undetected. These encouraging results have convinced us to utilize the pharmaceutical tool in daily practice.

The few "false-positive" cases identified helped improve and/or adapt the algorithms. This strengthens the need to implement a continuous improvement process, by updating recommendations, introducing new drugs and medications on the market, or revising biology standards. In addition, new algorithms were gradually developed and put into production. At the end of 2019, 13 automated algorithms were implemented at the CHU de Liège and used on a daily basis. Regular validation of the tool is recommended. The validation methodology, built in collaboration between hospital pharmacists, computer scientists and biostatisticians, served as a basis for future validations.

In practice, the alerts generated by the IT pharmaceutical tool are centrally collected and reviewed by hospital pharmacists attached to the CHU pharmacy department. The synergy between tools and pharmacists allows for the optimization of centralized pharmacotherapeutic management. The potential errors systematically highlighted by the tool and analyzed by a pharmacist allow for adequate interventions with a physician, and greatly contribute to improving the pharmacist–physician collaboration.

Although the overall specificity of 78% for the four algorithms tested was satisfactory, improvements are possible. The in-depth analysis of the prescriptions affected by the remaining 22% makes it possible to refine the algorithms. The CHU de Liège is also starting to reflect on the evaluation and improvement of patient file content, both as part of the JCI accreditation process and for the secondary purposes of clinical data exploitation. Actions that could be implemented in this context will help improve the pharmaceutical validation tool.

We noted from the literature that the medication error rate remains high for computerized systems linked with a basic CDSS arising from the large number of alerts generated, which contributes to the phenomenon of "fatigue alert", whereby the attention of clinicians decreases when faced with too many security alerts (AHRQ 2019). The alerts generated by the CHU tool are reviewed in depth by pharmacists and only lead to an intervention by a physician in a limited number of cases for the four algorithms tested, thereby reducing the phenomenon of "fatigue alert". Moreover, the high acceptance rate (81%) of pharmaceutical interventions by prescribing physicians is encouraging. We hope to see this rate increase further thanks to the recent establishment of a system of notes visible to all the doctors involved in patient care. So, for example, if the prescribing doctor is on call next day, the doctor replacing them will also able to see the intervention electronically.

Even if not precisely quantified, it is clear that the use of the tool achieved a time saving of more than 50% for the pharmacist in charge of the prescriptions. Finally, the targeted and automated tool installed meets the requested criterion that is part of the JCI accreditation process. Its development is therefore central to the institutional strategy.

4.5. References

AFSSAPS (2009). Guichet des erreurs médicamenteuses : présentation et bilan depuis la mise en place. Assessment, AFSSAPS, France.

AHRQ (2019). Alert fatigue. Agency for Healthcare Research and Quality (AHRQ) [Online]. Available at: https://psnet.ahrq.gov/primer/alert-fatigue [Accessed 23 May 2019].

Durand, D. (2012). La prise en charge des erreurs médicamenteuses à l'ANSM. *ANSM*, France.

JCI (2017). Medication management and use. In *Joint Commission International Accreditation Standards for Hospitals*, 6th edition, Joint Commission International (ed.). Oak Brook, IL.

Mahé, J. (2014). Erreurs médicamenteuses : définition, fréquence et gestion du risque. *La lettre du pharmacologue*, 28(1).

Seidling, H. and Bates, D.W. (2016). Evaluating the impact of health IT on medication safety. *Studies in Health Technology and Informatics*, 222, 195–205.

Streel, S. (2019). Mise en place et validation d'un outil automatisé et ciblé d'analyse pharmaceutique au CHU de Liège. Thesis, CHU de Liège, Belgium.

5

Simulation of Countermeasures in the Face of Covid-19 Using a Linear Compartmental Model

5.1. Introduction

Our community is facing a pandemic, which has led to the confinement of over half the inhabitants of our planet. We are disarmed in the face of the coronavirus (SARS-CoV-2), and lockdown measures seem to be the only countermeasure capable of containing the pandemic, despite the resulting economic cost. The first works published focus on the characteristics of the disease (Cheng *et al.* 2020; Van der Werf and Peltekian 2020; Wang *et al.* 2020), on the contagiousness of the disease (Liu *et al.* 2020; Rocklöv *et al.* 2020; Yuan *et al.* 2020), on possible first-line treatments (Chen *et al.* 2020; Gautret *et al.* 2020; HCSP 2020), on intensive care units (ICUs) (Azoulay *et al.* 2020; Darmon *et al.* 2020; Ministère de la Santé 2020; Schultz *et al.* 2020) and on containment (Gram Pedersen and Meneghin 2020; Rocklöv *et al.* 2020). We did not find any articles dealing with the simulation of the Covid-19 pandemic for the purpose of evaluating and scaling medical countermeasures.

The SIR (Susceptible–Infected–Recovered) model is known in epidemiology as a compartmental model. The SIR model, in its basic formulation, stratifies the population into three health states: susceptible to the disease (noted S), infected with the disease (noted I) and recovered from the disease (noted R). In many cases in the literature, infected persons are detailed in several states: *latent* (i.e. without symptoms), *prodromal* (i.e. with symptoms) and *fulminant* (i.e. in a severe/deteriorated state) (Perra and Gonçalves 2015, pp. 59–83; Guinet *et al.* 2018).

Chapter written by Alain GUINET.

In order to simulate the epidemic, we use this framework as a flow model, calculating the people in different stages of the disease and under different medical treatments by period and propagating the flows of people between states by period. We use a discrete representation of the SIR model over a horizon of daily periods. When the disease is not transmitted directly from person to person (e.g. a case of poisoning) or when the infection rate is constant for an entire population (e.g. seasonal influenza), the SIR model can be linearized (Guinet *et al.* 2018; Liu *et al.* 2019). The transmission rate from S to I is assumed to be constant and the propagation of the flow from S to I can be approximated according to S. Perra and Gonçalves (2015, pp. 59–83) propose to calculate the rate of β propagation from S to I as a function of a demographically adapted function λ such that $\lambda = \beta * I$, where λ represents the force of the infection. The latter is equal to the probability of being infected multiplied by the number of contacts. Knowing the basic reproduction number $R0$ (Guerra *et al.* 2017), which is equal to the probability of being infected multiplied by the number of contacts multiplied by the duration of contagion D, as well as I the number of infected people, we can calculate the rate of propagation β. The number of people infected assumes that all symptomatic and asymptomatic cases are known.

In the case of the Diamond Princess cruise ship, which was infected with a single case of Covid-19, all the passengers were tested for the disease and all symptomatic and asymptomatic patients are known (Mizumoto and Chowell 2020; Rocklöv *et al.* 2020). In this cluster, the population living on the ship is, of course, more homogeneous, compared to the more disparate population of Wuhan or France. Thanks to Rocklöv *et al.* (2020), the basic reproduction number $R0$ for the disease is available. β is therefore equal to $R0/(D * I)$, where I is considered as a scale factor. In addition, the passengers of the Diamond Princess cruise ship have been confined to the ship in an effort to stop the disease by reducing the number of contacts, in order to lower the base reproduction number $R0$ and reducing it to $R1$.

5.2. The compartmental model

5.2.1. *Model assumptions*

In Figure 5.1, an individual first appears in the susceptible state (S). They become infected if they acquire the disease (I). If symptoms appear, they reach the prodromal state (P). If treatment is available, the patient receives first-line treatment in a hospital (T). If left untreated or if treatment fails, the patient goes into a fulminating state (F). They can then be admitted to an available intensive care bed (C). Finally, they either recover (R) after hospitalization in post-intensive care (H) or die (D).

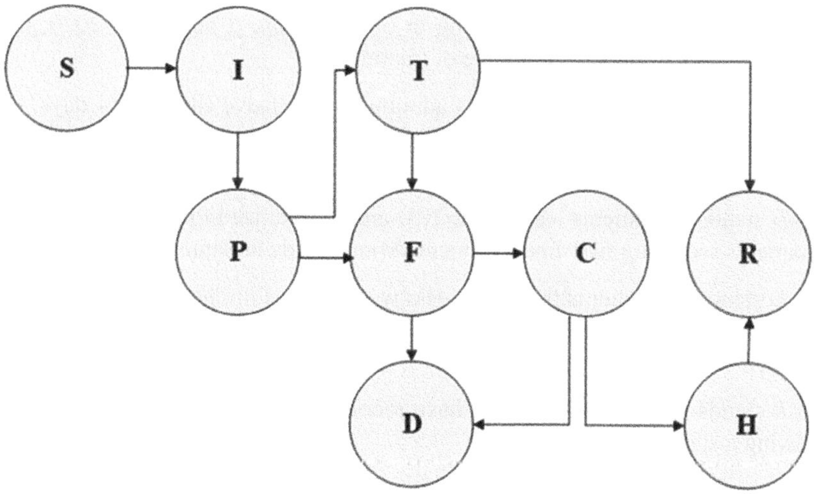

Figure 5.1. *The compartmental model*

5.2.2. *Model parameters*

More precisely, the states of the compartmental model are:

– *S* stands for susceptible, that is, patients who may be infected;

– *I* stands for infected, that is, patients with the Covid-19 disease; either $R0 = 4.8$ without confinement (Roques *et al.*, 2020) or $R1 = 1.78$ with confinement (Rocklöv *et al.* 2020), $D = 20$ (Roques *et al.* 2020), I = 621 (Mizumoto and Chowell 2020) and the propagation rates from *S* to *I* are $\beta 0 = 4.8/(20 * 621) \approx 0.0386\%$ and $\beta 1 = 1.78/(20 * 621) \approx 0.0143\%$, respectively;

– *P* stands for prodromal, that is, those infected patients who develop symptoms after an average incubation period of 6 days (Yuan *et al.* 2020), the rate of spread from *I* to *P* is equal to 30% (Darmon *et al.* 2020; Mizumoto and Chowell 2020; Rocklöv *et al.* 2020);

– *T* stands for patients on first-line treatment (e.g. antiviral, anti-inflammatory, antibiotic treatments) (Chen *et al.* 2020; Gautret *et al.* 2020; HCSP 2020), that is, prodromal patients treated as early as the onset of symptoms for a period of 10 days (Darmon *et al.* 2020);

– *F* stands for fulminating patients, that is, those infected and in acute respiratory distress, who are hospitalized in the emergency room and awaiting an intensive care bed with mechanical ventilation; prodromal patients become fulminant patients if they are not treated with first-line therapy; patients who are resistant to first-line treatment become fulminant with a rate equal to 21% (Santé Publique France 2020) or with a rate equal to 5% according to other authors (Chen *et al.* 2020; Gautret *et al.* 2020) depending on the choice of treatment;

– C stands for fulminant patients admitted to intensive care for 14 days, that is, fulminant patients who obtained one of the 15,000 beds (Ministère de la Santé 2020);

– H stands for patients leaving the ICU and hospitalized for a further 10 days and the patients receiving first-line treatment (Ministère de la Santé 2020);

– D stands for patients that died, who were either fulminating and did not find a bed in an ICU (100%) or died in an ICU (37%) (Annane *et al.* 2012; Ministère de la Santé 2020);

– R stands for the patients who have recovered following first-line treatment or following a stay in an ICU.

5.3. A linear SIR model

A linear model is proposed for simulation purposes, we specify its data, its variables, its objective function and its constraints.

5.3.1. *Data*

– Nbstat: the number of patient states. Nine states are defined (S for susceptible, I for infected, P for prodromal, T for under first-line treatment, F for fulminant, C for hospitalized in intensive care units, H for hospitalized, R for recovered, D for deceased);

– Nper: the number of periods in days (a horizon of 180 days is studied);

– Nepat: the number of people likely to be infected, that is, the French population or the population in the AURA (Auvergne Rhône-Alpes) region;

– Irat: the infection rate, that is, the percentage of susceptible persons infected without confinement, that is, 0.0386%;

– Icnf: the infection rate, that is, the percentage of susceptible persons infected with confinement, that is, 0.0143%;

– Prat: the prodromal rate, that is, percentage of people developing symptoms, 30%;

– Frat: the failure rate of first-line treatments, 21% or 5%;

– Crat: the ICU treatment failure rate, 37%;

– Drat: the death rate, that is, percentage of people who died awaiting intensive care, 100%;

– Canti: the cost of first-line treatment in a hospital per day, €1,200;

– Cicu: the cost of the patient's stay in intensive care, €2,300;

– Hlife: the estimated cost of a human life in terms of legal compensation in France for a victim aged 65, that is, €300,000 according to ONIAM (https://www.oniam.fr/procedure-indemnisation/bareme-indemnisation); a cost in human life allows us to avoid multi-criteria optimization (Guinet *et al.* 2018);

– Nbed: the number of intensive care beds available to receive patients;

– Nmed: the number of facilities available to receive patients for medical services;

– CHdose: the number of first-line treatments available (1,000,000);

– Cdet: the period for the start of confinement, it extends until the end of the epidemic;

– Pdet: the period for the end of the epidemic (an assumption of seasonality is considered);

– Alos: the length of hospitalization in a medical department for first-line treatment, that is, 10 days;

– Ilos: the length of hospitalization in an ICU, that is, 14 days;

– Hlos: the length of hospitalization in a medical service after ICU, that is, 10 days;

– Lin: the incubation period, that is, 6 days.

5.3.2. *Variables*

– EVs(p): the number of people who enter a state $s = \{S, I, P, T, F, C, H, D, R\}$ at the start of period p.

5.3.3. *Objective function*

$$Minimize\ (Z) = \sum_{p=1}^{Nper} EVD(p) * Hlife + \sum_{p=1}^{Nper} EVC(p) * Cicu * Ilos + \sum_{p=1}^{Nper} EVT(p) * Canti * Alos + \sum_{p=1}^{Nper} EVH(p) * Canti * Hlos \qquad [5.1]$$

The costs of medical responses are minimized, that is, the cost of compensating the deceased, the cost of first-line treatment and the cost of intensive care. As the cost of compensation is at least 10 times higher than the other costs, minimizing the number of deaths is thus a major criterion.

5.3.4. *Constraints*

$$EVS(1) = Nepat \quad [5.2a]$$

$$EVS(p) = EVS(p-1) * (1 - Irat) \quad p = 2, \ldots, Cdet - 1 \quad [5.2b]$$

$$EVS(p) = EVS(p-1) * (1 - Icnf) \quad p = Cdet, \ldots, Pdet \quad [5.2c]$$

$$EVS(p) = 0 \quad p = Pdet + 1, \ldots, Nper \quad [5.2d]$$

People can be infected from the first period to the end of the epidemic (state *S*) according to different forces and dependent on containment.

$$EVI(p) = 0 \quad p = 1, \ldots, Lin \quad [5.3a]$$

$$EVI(p) = EVS(p - lin) * Irat \quad p = Lin + 1, \ldots, Cdet - 1 \quad [5.3b]$$

$$EVI(p) = EVS(p - lin) * Icnf \quad p = Cdet, \ldots, Nper \quad [5.3c]$$

People in contact are infected and are symptomatic or asymptomatic after Lin days of incubation (state *I*).

$$EVP(p) = 0 \quad p = 1, \ldots, Lin \quad [5.4a]$$

$$EVP(p) = EVI(p-1) * Prat - EVT(p-1)$$

$$p = Lin + 1, \ldots, Nper \quad [5.4b]$$

Some people develop symptoms (state *P*). First-line treatments are administered as soon as symptoms appear (state *T*).

$$EVT(p) = 0 \quad p = 1, \ldots, Lin \quad [5.5a]$$

$$\sum_{p=Lin}^{Nper} EVT(p) \leq CHdose \quad [5.5b]$$

The number of first-line treatments is limited.

$$EVF(p) = 0 \quad p = 1, \ldots, Lin \quad [5.6a]$$

$$EVF(p) = EVF(p-1) * (1 - Drat) + EVP(p-1) - EVC(p-1)$$

$$p = Lin + 1, \dots, Lin + Alos \qquad [5.6b]$$

$$EVFp = EVF(p-1) * (1 - Drat) + EVP(p-1) - EVC(p-1)$$

$$+ EVT(p-1) * Frat$$

$$p = Lin + Alos + 1, \dots, Nper \qquad [5.6c]$$

After Lin days of incubation without treatment, patients are waiting to be hospitalized into intensive care units (state *F*), a portion of whom are admitted (state *C*) and a portion who die due to a lack of beds. Patients who are resistant to first-line treatment also become fulminant.

$$EVC(p) = 0 \quad p = 1, \dots, Lin \qquad [5.7a]$$

$$\sum_{q=p}^{p+Ilos-1} EVC(q) \leq Nbed \quad p = 1, \dots, Nper - Ilos + 1 \qquad [5.7b]$$

The number of ICU beds is limited for each period. Patients admitted to the ICU from period p to (p + *ILos-1*) will occupy a bed during Ilos periods, that is, their length of stay. The bed capacity must be checked for each period of the stay.

$$EVH(p) = 0 \quad p = 1, \dots, Lin + Ilos - 1 \qquad [5.8a]$$

$$EVH(p + Ilos) = EVC(p) * (1 - Crat)$$

$$p = Lin, \dots, Nper - Ilos \qquad [5.8b]$$

The stay in medical care follows the stay in intensive care (state *H*) Ilos periods later.

$$\sum_{q=p}^{p+Hlos-1} EVH(q) + \sum_{q=p}^{P+Alos-1} EVT(q) \leq Nmed$$

$$p = Lin, \dots, Nper - Max[Hlos, Alos] + 1 \qquad [5.9]$$

The number of medical facilities are limited and are used for a defined period of stay. We calculate the number of patients from period p to period (p + *Hlos-1*) or (*P* + *Alos*) with the knowledge that these last two terms are constants.

$$EVD(p) = 0 \quad p = 1, \dots, Lin \qquad [5.10a]$$

$$EVD(p) = EVF(p-1) * Drat + EVC(p-1) * Crat$$

$$p = Lin, \dots, Nper \qquad [5.10b]$$

The untreated people and patients who are in ICU and died (state *D*).

$$EVR(p) = 0 \quad p = 1, \dots, Lin \tag{5.11a}$$

$$EVR(p) = EVI(p-1) * (1 - Prat)$$

$$p = Lin + 1, \dots, Lin + Alos \tag{5.11b}$$

$$EVR(p) = EVI(p-1) * (1 - Prat) + EVT(p - Alos) * (1 - Frat)$$

$$p = Lin + Alos + 1, \dots, Lin + Min(Alos, Hlos) + Ilos \tag{5.11c}$$

$$EVR(p) = EVI(p-1) * (1 - Prat) + EVT(p - Alos) * (1 - Frat)$$

$$+EVC(p - Ilos - Hlos) * (1 - Crat)$$

$$p = Lin + Min(Alos, Hlos) + Ilos + 1, \dots, Nper \tag{5.11d}$$

The people who recovered, or are asymptomatic, together with those patients who were cured by first-line treatment or in an ICU (state *R*).

5.4. Results

We are studying the period from February 23 to May 23, 2020, that is, a 90-day horizon. The confinement of the population began on March 17, which is day 22. Problems are resolved with Cplex[1]. The parameters of the model are defined in one Excel sheet, and the results are written in another Excel sheet. Confinement countermeasures versus the effectiveness of possible first-line treatments are simulated. The failure rate of first-line treatment is 21% or 5%, depending on the authors.

Regarding the victims, our results are fairly close to the reality to which we have sadly borne witness (28,367 deaths on May 24 for France and 2,702 deaths on May 14 for the AURA region), with the knowledge that these were very roughly approximated (see Tables 5.1 and 5.2) and that deaths in the model go beyond May 24. An effective first-line treatment, if it exists, seems to be the best countermeasure in the fight against the Covid-19 pandemic, drastically reducing the number of deaths, that is, dividing it by 5. However, the confinement of inhabitants is also a simple and effective countermeasure, in effect, reducing the number of victims by half. Regarding the use of intensive care beds, effective first-line treatment is an efficient countermeasure, reducing the strain on medical resources by 3. Calculation times are approximately 3 seconds for each scenario. The Cplex model developed is available on request.

1 Available at: https://www.ibm.com/search?lang=en&cc=us&q=Cplex.

Scenarios for France	Number of people infected	Number of people treated	Number of people in ICU	Number of deaths	Number of recoveries	Cost of the medical response in K€
With containment	1,065,949	319,785	60,054	**29,320**	1,036,629	15,021,423
With containment + effective treatment	1,065,949	319,785	15,989	5,916	1,060,033	6,247,955
Without confinement	2,115,408	634,622	93,406	74,425	2,040,983	33,656,811
Without containment + effective treatment	2,115,408	634,622	31,731	11,741	2,103,667	12,399,250

Table 5.1. *Scenarios for mainland France (65 million inhabitants)*

Scenarios for AURA region	Number of people infected	Number of people treated	Number of people in ICU	Number of deaths	Number of recoveries	Cost of the medical response in K€
With containment	131,194	39,358	8,265	**3,058**	128,136	1,718,360
With containment + effective treatment	131,194	39,358	1,968	728	130,466	768,979
Without confinement	260,358	78,107	16,403	6,069	254,289	3,410,136
Without containment + effective treatment	260,358	78,107	3,905	1,445	258,913	1,526,061

Table 5.2. *Scenarios for the AURA region (8 million inhabitants)*

5.5. Conclusion

We have studied the effectiveness of the health countermeasure adopted by half of the countries of the world as a means of dealing with the Covid-19 pandemic. Containment of the population seems to be a well-suited action in the absence of an effective treatment, such as a viral treatment or a vaccine. In France, the confinement of the population did not have exactly the same impact on the AURA region as it did on the whole country. In the event of a second wave, more specific confinements that make an assessment by region, by department or by city may be more appropriate.

5.6. References

Annane, D., Diehl, J.-L., Drault, J.-N., Farkas, J.-C., Gouello, J.-P., Fourrier, F., Fraïsse, F., Jars-Guincestre, M.-C., Mira, J.-P., Misset, B., Outin, H., Monnet, X., Reignier, J., Souweine, B., Thevenin, D., Vieillard-Baron, A., Wolff, M. (2012). Démographie et structures des services de réanimation français (hors réanimation chirurgicale) : état des lieux. *Réanimation*, 21, S540–S561.

Azoulay, E., Beloucif, S., Vivien, B., Guidet, B., Pateron, D., Le Dorze, M. (2020). Décision d'admission des patients en unités de réanimation et unités de soins critiques dans un contexte d'épidémie à Covid-19 [Online]. Available at: https://www.srlf.org/wp-content/uploads/2020/03/ARS-ETHIQUE-COVID-final.pdf.

Chen, Z., Hu, J., Zhang, Z., Jiang, S., Han, S., Yan, D., Zhuang, R., Hu, B., Zhang, Z. (2020). Efficacy of hydroxychloroquine in patients with COVID-19: Results of a randomized clinical trial. *MedRxiv* [Online]. Available at: https://www.medrxiv.org/content/10.1101/2020.03.22.20040758v3.full.pdf+html.

Cheng, Z., Yu, T., Xia, J., Wei, Y., Wu, W., Xie, X., Yin, W., Li, H., Liu, M., Xiao, Y., Gao, H., Guo, L., Xie, J., Wang, G., Jiang, R., Gao, Z., Jin, Q., Wang, J., Cao, B. (2020). Clinical features of patients infected with 2019 novel coronavirus in Wuhan, China. *The Lancet*, 395, 497–506

Darmon, M., Bouadma, L., Morawiec, E., Constantin, J.-M., Montravers, P., Zahar, J.-R., Lucet, J.-C., Guery, B., Bessis, S., Saidani, N., Renolleau, S. (2020). Recommandations d'experts portant sur la prise en charge en réanimation des patients en période d'épidémie à SARS-CoV2 [Online]. Available at: https://sfar.org/recommandations-dexperts-portant-sur-la-prise-en-charge-en-reanimation-des-patients-en-periode-depidemie-a-sars-cov2/.

Gautret, P., Lagier, J.-C., Parola, P., Thuan Hoang, V., Meddeb, L., Sevestre, J., Mailhe, M., Doudier, B., Aubry, C., Amrane, S., Seng, P., Hocquart, M., Eldin, C., Finance, J., Esteves Vieira, V., Tissot Dupont, H., Honoré, S., Stein, A., Million, M., Colson, P., La Scola, B., Veit, V., Jacquier, A., Deharo, J.-C., Drancourt, M., Fournier, P.-E., Rolain, J.-M., Brouqui, P., Raoult, D. (2020). Clinical and microbiological effect of a combination of hydroxychloroquine and azithromycin in 80 COVID-19 patients with at least a six-day follow up: An observational study. *Travel Medicine and Infectious Disease*, 34, 101663.

Giordano, G., Blanchini, F., Bruno, R., Colaneri, P., Di Filippo, A., Di Matteo, A., Colaneri, M., COVID19 IRCCS San Matteo Pavia Task Force (2020). A SIDARTHE model of COVID-19 epidemic in Italy [Online]. Available at: https://arxiv.org/pdf/2003.09861.pdf.

Gram Pedersen, M. and Meneghin, M. (2020). Quantifying undetected COVID-19 cases and effects of containment measures in Italy: Predicting phase 2 dynamics. Paper [Online]. Available at: https://www.researchgate.net/publication/339915690_Quantifying_undetected_COVID-19_cases_and_effects_of_containment_measures_in_Italy_Predicting_phase_2_dynamics.

Guerra, F., Bolotin, S., Lim, G., Heffernan, J., Deeks, S., Li, Y., Crowcroft, N. (2017). The basic reproduction number (R0) of measles: A systematic review. *The Lancet*, 17, 420–428.

Guinet, A., Barkaoui, H., Wang, T., Dubost, E. (2018). An emergency management plan to face a foodborne criminal attack. *7th International Conference on Information Systems, Logistics and Supply Chain (ILS 2018)*, Lyon, France, 8–11 July.

HCSP (2020). Avis relatif aux recommandations thérapeutiques dans la prise en charge du COVID-19 [Online]. Available at: https://sfar.org/download/avis-relatif-aux-recommandations-therapeutiques-dans-la-prise-en-charge-du-covid-19/?wpdmdl=25647&refresh=5e7cadbce4e901585229244.

Liu, M., Xu, X., Cao, J., Zhang, D. (2019). Integrated planning for public health emergencies: A modified model for controlling H1N1 pandemic. *Journal of the Operational Research Society*, 71(5), 748–761.

Liu, Y., Gayle, A., Wilder-Smith, A., Rocklöv, J. (2020). The reproductive number of COVID-19 is higher compared to SARS coronavirus. *Journal of Travel Medicine*, 27(2), 1–4.

Ministère de la santé (2020). Besoins en réanimation et réponse capacitaire. Recommandations aux établissements de santé. Recommendations, 22 March.

Mizumoto, K. and Chowell, G. (2020). Transmission potential of the novel coronavirus (COVID-19) onboard the Diamond Princess cruise ship. *Infectious Disease Modelling*, 5, 264–270.

Perra, N. and Gonçalves, B. (2015). Modeling and predicting human infectious diseases. In *Social Phenomena*, Gonçalves, B. and Perra, N. (eds). Springer, Cham.

Rocklöv, J., Sjödin, H., Wilder-Smith, A. (2020). COVID-19 outbreak on the Diamond Princess cruise ship: Estimating the epidemic potential and effectiveness of public health countermeasures. *Journal of Travel Medicine*, 27, 1–7.

Roques, L., Klein, E.K., Papaïx, J., Sar, A., Soubeyrand, S. (2020). Using early data to estimate the actual infection fatality ratio from COVID-19 in France. *Biology*, 97, 1–10.

Santé Publique France (2020). COVID-19 Point épidémiologique hebdomadaire du 16 avril 2020. National bulletin, Santé Publique France.

Schultz, P., Morvan, J.-B., Fakhry, N., Morinière, S., Vergez, S., Lacroix, C., Bartier Beatrix Barry, S., Babin, E., Couloigner, V., Atallah, I. (2020). Consensus français sur la réalisation de trachéotomies et les soins de trachéotomies pendant la pandémie de COVID-19. *Annales françaises d'oto-rhino-laryngologie et de pathologie cervicofaciale*, 137(3), 158–160.

Tan, X., Yuan, L., Zhou, J., Zheng, Y., Yang, F. (2013). Modeling the initial transmission dynamics of influenza A H1N1 in Guangdong Province, China. *International Journal of Infectious Diseases*, 17, 479–484.

Van der Werf, S. and Peltekian, C. (2020). Émergence du coronavirus SARS-CoV-2 : faire face à l'épidémie de Covid-19. *Virologie*, 24(S1), S3–S6.

Wang, L., Wang, Y., Ye, D., Liu, Q. (2020). Review of the 2019 novel coronavirus (SARS-CoV-2) based on current evidence. *International Journal of Antimicrobial Agents*, 55(6), 105948.

Yuan, J., Li, M., Lv, G., Lv, Z.K. (2020). Monitoring transmissibility and mortality of COVID-19 in Europe. *International Journal of Infectious Diseases*, 95, 311–315.

PART 2

Digital and New Technologies for Health Services

Summary of Contributions – Part 2

Towards a New Classification of Medical Procedures in Belgium, *by Pol LECLERCQ, Sarah BARDIAUX, Djohra AZZI, Julie VAN DEN BULCKE and Magali PIRSON*

After years of hesitancy, Belgium is embarking on a structural reform of the nomenclature for medical procedures on the basis of a plan proposed by the *Département d'Economie de la Santé* (Department of Health Economics) of the *Université Libre de Bruxelles* or DESULB. The *Institut National d'Assurance Maladie Invalidité* (National Institute of Health and Disability Insurance) or *INAMI* coordinates the first phase of the reform aimed at modernizing the descriptive part of the nomenclature in order to have a classification described by standardized and precise wording. This contribution concerns the standardization and classification of medical-surgical technical procedures. It describes the steps necessary for the implementation of this classification through the mobilization of three categories of medical experts: (1) an expert in medical classification; (2) doctors recognized in their disciplines for medical pre-validation; and (3) groups of experts from the various specialties chosen by INAMI, responsible for validating the standardization work.

Digital Toolkit for the Ergonomic Evaluation of Workstations, *by Valentin ROCHAT and Antoine HAYEK.*

Thanks to the introduction of information technologies, scientific methods and the mass of available data, health and healthcare centers will soon be able to prevent, anticipate, monitor and follow the evolution of public health in order to intervene at the right time with the right tools. In this context, ergonomics will increasingly occupy a place within these health and healthcare centers to carry out tasks such as the placement and handling of patients, the putting of meal trays on trolleys, all the while preserving the well-being of caregivers in their professional environment. This contribution presents examples of tools and services offered by ProcSim in the healthcare sector to provide solutions in terms of flows and processes in the context of digital transformation. It also presents the applied ergonomic evaluation process.

Simulation on an RFID Interactive Tabletop with Tangible Objects of Future Working Conditions: Prospects for Implementation in the Hospital Sector, *by Yoann LEBRUN, Nicolas VISPI, Sophie LEPREUX, Sondès CHAABANE and Christophe KOLSKI.*

In a changing world in which technologies evolve rapidly, health and healthcare systems must adapt, reorganize and transform. It is therefore essential that methods be put in place so that employees, whatever their profile, can be trained and can implement the new working conditions. To this end, this chapter proposes an interactive tabletop simulator equipped with the RFID technology that is associated with tangible objects. This simulator allows employees, such as caregivers, to see themselves in new situations in a collective framework around the interactive table. Different scenarios can be identified, set up and then replayed to facilitate this projection. A simulator based on the principle of interactive game-learning through scenarios allows for many perspectives in the hospital sector to be presented.

Robotic Geriatric Assistant: A Pilot Assessment in a Real-World Hospital, *by Dimitri VOILMY, Karine LAN HING TING, Ana IGLESIAS, Rebeca MARFIL, Juan Pedro BANDERA, Fernando FERNANDEZ and Quitterie DE ROLL.*

In the context of an aging population, the assessment and monitoring of elderly patients contributes to the objectives for the prevention and treatment of geriatric problems, namely to extend life span without disability and to preserve autonomy. The comprehensive geriatric assessment (CGA) is a multidimensional and multidisciplinary diagnostic instrument that allows personalized care to be offered to the elderly, based on the assessment of their state of health. This assessment is based on a vast collection of data on the medical, psychosocial and functional disabilities of the vulnerable elderly person, in order to develop a coordinated plan promoting healthy aging. However, due to a lack of sufficient resources, a large proportion of the vulnerable elderly population is currently receiving insufficient care or none at all. This contribution therefore describes a pilot assessment that was carried out with a geriatric robot assistant named Clara, allowing for the identification and monitoring of a greater number of elderly people, thus facilitating their care and improving their living conditions.

Perspectives on the Patient Experience (PX) of People with Disabilities in the Digital Age: From UX to PX, *by Djilali IDOUGHI, Karim TOULOUM, Yohan GUERRIER and Christophe KOLSKI.*

With the advent of digital and associated technologies aimed at transforming practices and applications within the health sector at large, and in particular healthcare delivery, the patient is now at the center of any modern healthcare system and often followed by several health professionals typically based in multiple locations. People with disabilities are particularly affected by this context and each person therefore has specific needs in relation to the systems in existence. For example, a blind person will not have the same needs as an upper or lower limb amputee. Therefore, it is important to take into account the general User eXperience (UX), and the Patient eXperience (PX), in particular. This contribution thus deals with the dimension of the digitization of care delivery aimed at a patient experience involving a disability. This refers in part to the Web Accessibility Initiative (WAI) as online services can help improve healthcare delivery.

6

Towards a New Classification of Medical Procedures in Belgium

6.1. Introduction

6.1.1. *An essential but obsolete medical healthcare nomenclature*

In Belgium, the *Nomenclature des Prestations de Santé* or NPS (i.e. Nomenclature of Medical Procedures) is an essential tool for funding physicians and hospitals. In addition to this main application, NPS records are used by institutions for the planning and budgeting of medical resources, for epidemiological and economic studies and for the transmission of information to international authorities (Eurostat, OECD, etc.).

Over the last 50 years, the NPS has been adapted, however its basic structure has never been completely redesigned. It thus appears as a disparate set of chapters with no order. Over time, criticisms have multiplied: lack of transparency in the development of tariffs, inter- and intra-disciplinary inequalities, obsolete or missing procedures, imprecision in the formulation of medical procedures leading to questionable interpretations.

In 1993, the Minister of Social Affairs commissioned two universities to conduct a broad international review of the methods for determining medical fees. The objective was to readjust the NPS tariffs based on "scientific" criteria. The studies and proposals (Devillé *et al.* 1993; Leclercq *et al.* 1996) attracted interest from physicians, but the project was abandoned by the new minister. Since then, several initiatives have followed one another without success due to a lack of political will in the face of the scope of such a reform.

Chapter written by Pol LECLERCQ, Sarah BARDIAUX, Djohra AZZI, Julie VAN DEN BULCKE and Magali PIRSON.

During studies on the cost of certain medical procedures, carried out at the request of the Minister of Social Affairs in 2016–2017 (Leclercq and Pirson 2018), our Department of Health Economics (DESULB) noted that the professionals consulted (physicians, nurses, technicians) regularly came up against a lack of clarity in the wording describing a number of medical provisions. As many actions or techniques were combined in a single formulation, the application of cost calculation methods would, in some cases, lose relevance because they were too approximate. It was obvious that the very structure of the nomenclature needed to be revised. In short, an updated and standardized descriptive classification of the nomenclature should precede a reform of the tariffs.

6.1.2. *Decision to initiate a structural reform of the Belgian healthcare nomenclature*

In March 2019, at the request of the *Institut National d'Assurance Maladie Invalidité* or INAMI (the Belgian National Institute of Health and Disability Insurance), responsible for the nomenclature of healthcare, DESULB[1] was asked to present a framework plan for the structural reform of the health care nomenclature, NPS V0[2] (Leclercq and Pirson 2019). The project was accepted by the *Commission Nationale Médico Mutuelliste* (CNMM[3]), which allowed INAMI to implement the realization of a first phase of the reform as of June 1, 2019.

The study would be conducted in three phases:

1) standardization of formulations and classification of medical procedures;

2) adjustment of professional fee rates;

3) establishment of rates for operating costs related to medical activity.

The duration of the first phase of the reform was set at 24 months[4]. The pricing studies of the second and third phases necessarily imply that the formulations of the procedures that are the subject of the studies have been standardized beforehand to provide the degree of precision that is essential for the "pricing" phases.

1 DESULB is the term used throughout this chapter to represent the association of two research centers: CR1ESPULB, GEDIS.

2 NPS V0 is the agreed upon acronym to designate the Belgian nomenclature of medical procedures in its current form.

3 CNMM: The National-Medico-Mutualist Commission is the body of INAMI. where tariffs are negotiated between insurance companies and the representatives of the medical unions.

4 24 months would allow a first standardization but it would still take another 6 to 12 months to finalize the common classification which will mark the final completion of Phase 1 (see section 6.2 methodologies).

Even though the methodologies for subsequent steps (2) and (3) have already been presented in the framework plan, they still need to be discussed in further detail. The duration of the work leading to new tariffs is estimated to be between 36 and 48 months.

These studies will require the unbundling of professional fees and operating costs that are currently tightly integrated into a *global fee*[5] for most NPS V0 procedures.

6.1.3. *The NPS V0 nomenclature in a few figures*

As of 2018, the NPS V0 included approximately 7,556 tariff descriptions of all types (fixed prices, tariffs for paramedical services, dental services, medical procedures, etc.). It is used to transfer the budget for health and disability insurance, that is, 29 billion euros to healthcare providers (hospitals, physicians and other healthcare professionals). The planned reform concerns the 3,913 medical procedures.

For the first phase (descriptive classification), it would be difficult to apply a single standardization method to all 3,913 medical procedures. These were divided into three categories: (a) biology, genetics, anatomical pathology, radiotherapy, numbering 895 (AMTA); (b) consultations, advice and similar services, numbering 345 (ACA) and (c) all other medical and surgical technical procedures (ATMC) numbering 2,673. Each category will be the subject of specific approaches adapted to the nature of the services grouped therein.

Through the reform of the nomenclature, INAMI is mainly seeking to rebalance the average incomes of physicians in the various specialties. In this perspective, the different specific approaches leading to a "pricing" nomenclature (Phases 2 and 3) will have to be closely coordinated.

6.1.4. *Purpose of the presentation*

The presentation focuses on the standardization and classification of 2,673 medico-surgical technical procedures (ATMC). A review of the literature shows that there is a wealth of documentation on the classification of medical procedures.

---

5 In Belgian parlance, a "pure" or "professional" fee is used when the tariff sets the amount that is intended solely for the physician's fee. When the fee is "global", it covers both the physician's remuneration and the cost of the practice. In a hospital, if the physician is self-employed (which is generally the case in Belgium), the hospital manager and the physician (or their representatives) must agree on the percentage of the fee that will be retroceded and the amount that will be acquired by the hospital to cover the operating costs inherent in performing the procedure. This distribution is the result of a negotiation that varies from hospital to hospital.

However, there are few articles describing the steps taken to arrive at these classifications. When faced with such a project (modernizing an obsolete nomenclature), we look for all the national or regional experiences that could serve as a model, even if each development reflects its own context and particularities.

6.2. Methodology

If the final objective is to achieve a common classification of medical procedures, then it is necessary to work with specialists from the various medico-surgical disciplines to standardize and classify these services. In this respect, there is a tendency towards over-specialization, which complicates the dialogue and multiplies the number of interlocutors. The 2,673 ATMCs in the current NPS V0 nomenclature have been produced by around 30 medical specialties or sub-specialties. During the standardization process, certain specialties were “split up” into sub-specialties. This was the case with thoracic surgery or orthopedic surgery. This could still be the case with abdominal surgery or medical imaging (Table 6.1.).

Disciplines	NPS V0	%	Disciplines	NPS V0	%
ENT	176	6.6%	Nephrology	11	0.4%
Cardiac surgery	37	1.4%	Physiotherapy	27	1.0%
Thoracic surgery	36	1.3%	Neurology	19	0.7%
Pneumology	34	1.3%	Neurosurgery	53	2.0%
Cardiology	54	2.0%	Spine surgery	203	7.6%
Urology	143	5.3%	Upper limb surgery	148	5.5%
Abdominal surgery	170	6.4%	Hand surgery	142	5.3%
OB-GYN	149	5.6%	Lower limb surgery	157	5.9%
Gastroenterology	68	2.5%	Foot surgery	136	5.1%
Plastic surgery	94	3.5%	Other orthopedic surgery	75	2.8%
Vascular surgery	75	2.8%	Anesthesiology	74	2.8%
Stomatology	141	5.3%	Imaging	215	8.0%
Ophtalmology	120	4.5%	Pediatrics	31	1.2%
Dermatology	32	1.2%	Rhumatology	7	0.3%
Hematology	17	0.6%	Other	29	1. 1%
			Total	2. 673	

Table 6.1. *NPS ATMC V0, medico-surgical technical procedures classified by specialty*

The 2,673 ATMCs of the NPS V0 were divided into six batches of +/– 450 denominations. Each batch is processed in five successive steps (Figure 6.1).

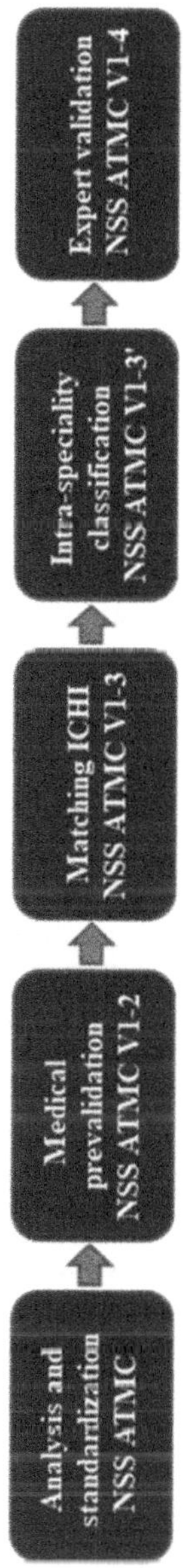

Figure 6.1. *The standardization and classification procedure*

The total processing time for a batch of +/– 450 ATMC is eight months, divided into two 4-month periods. The DESULB team must ensure the completion of the first four steps leading to a medically pre-validated standardization proposal for 450 formulations so that the full analysis and structuring of the 2,673 ATMCs is completed by May 31. INAMI is then supposed to continue onto the next stage within 4 months. In this schedule, the last batch of 450 ATMCs is expected to be definitively validated by September 30, 2021.

6.2.1. *Term analysis and standardization (NPS ATMC V1-1)*

A DESULB team comprising two university-trained, specialized nurses, supervised by two academic promoters (a physician, a nurse and a doctor in public health), carry out this first stage. The formulation of each ATMC is analyzed, broken down according to a triaxial logic (topography, action, means) and rewritten according to standardization rules (Leclercq *et al.* 2019) inspired by international classifications (CCAM 2001, ICHI, etc.). The result is an Excel table (Table 6.2.) containing, for each original service, all the information accumulated during the analysis process, the proposed new terms, the type of procedure, the notes and modifiers[6], the comments and questions raised.

6.2.2. *Medical pre-validation (NPS ATMC V1-2)*

Before transmitting the files to INAMI, the DESULB team arranges for its preliminary analysis and standardization work to be validated by medical specialists in each studied discipline. Two courses of action are initiated simultaneously:

(a) A consulting physician, an expert with 20 years' experience in the classification of medical procedures abroad, guided the DESULB team for several months by drawing the team's attention to what might constitute potential errors in syntax, consistency, precision or what would require further clarification. Gradually, DESULB members have acquired practical expertise.

---

6 Notes: to respect a principle of conciseness, the formulation of the term is limited to a strict description of the medical procedure. Additional information may be useful to explain certain terms or to indicate the conditions of use of the service. This information is attached in the form of notes that allow for correct interpretation of the formulation.

Modifiers: this is a category of billing rules that relate to the circumstances surrounding the performance of the procedure and which modify the reimbursement value (e.g. the age of the patient). The rules in this category must have common characteristics (they must relate to a patient characteristic that may affect the conditions under which the procedure is performed).

Hospit code	Formulation	Target	Action	Means	Hospit modified code	Formulation NSS ATMC V1-1	ETC
589201	percutaneous endovascular aortic valve surgery, a congenital malformation of the aorta, of the pulmonary valve, of the mitral valve, of the tricuspid valve or fulguration of a valve, including manipulations and controls during the treatment and the catheters used, excluding the dilation catheter(s) and pharmaceutical and contrast products, maximum per operating session	Aortic valve	Repair (plasty)	Percutaneous transluminal	589201a	percutaneous endovascular aortic valve plasty	
		Aortic arch / Aorta, thoracic descending	Repair (plasty)	Percutaneous transluminal	589201b	percutaneous endovascular congenital malformation of the aorta plasty	
		Pulmonary valve	Repair (plasty)	Percutaneous transluminal	589201c	percutaneous endovascular pulmonary valve plasty	
		Mitral valve	Repair (plasty)	Percutaneous transluminal	589201d	percutaneous endovascular mitral valve plasty	
		Tricuspid valve	Repair (plasty)	Percutaneous transluminal	589201e	percutaneous endovascular tricuspid valve plasty	
		Cardiac valve, unspecified	Fulguration	Percutaneous transluminal	589201f	percutaneous endovascular fulguration of a valve	

Table 6.2. *An example of pre-standardized terms prepared by DESULB*

(b) One or more physicians in charge of academic services with whom the DESULB team is used to collaborating, for example, in the 2016–2017 study cited above (Leclercq and Pirson 2018), are invited to answer unanswered questions, to discuss the appropriateness of a formulation, to modify and complete the preliminary work presented to them and commented on by the DESULB team. This medical pre-validation is unofficial since these experts have not been selected according to a procedure implemented by a public authority. For each specialty, there are between one and three sessions of two to four hours of work.

During this step (Table 6.3.), pre-validating physicians can:

– propose the deletion of ATMCs which, according to them are obsolete, no longer correspond to good medical practice or correspond to duplications in the nomenclature;

– propose the creation of new procedures because they do not exist in the nomenclature but are routinely performed (in this case, it is necessary to cite the assimilations most often used or to justify the proposal);

– modify one of the structuring axes, provide additional details or answer questions from the DESULB team. If necessary, the formulation will be rewritten (minor or major modification compared to the initial entry).

6.2.3. *Matching the WHO International Classification of Health Interventions (NPS ATMC V1-3)*

To facilitate international comparisons, each standardized formulation (NPS ATMC V1-2) is then matched with the similar axes of the ICHI[7] classification. To perform this operation, it is necessary to learn the coding rules for this classification (ICHI Beta-3 reference guide) and use the browser developed by WHO–FIC[8] (ICHI Platform User Guide). DESULB also uses the rating scale developed by the Nordic Center for Classifications in Healthcare (Almborg *et al.* 2017). This scale allows an assessment of the correlations between the axis for the classification of NPS ATMC V1-2 and the ICHI axis. The different scores, calculated according to the scale, correspond to different actions intended to harmonize the two classifications. At the end of this step, a correlation is established for each standardized formulation written in French and the ICHI classification (NPS ATMC V1-3) (Table 6.4.).

7 International Classification of Health Interventions.

8 WHO – Family of International Classifications.

	NSS ATMC V0	NSS ATMC V1-2					
Hospit code	Formulation	Target	Action	Means	Hospit modified code	Formulation NSS ATMC V1-1	ETC
589201	percutaneous endovascular aortic valve surgery, a congenital malformation of the aorta, of the pulmonary valve, of the mitral valve, of the tricuspid valve or fulguration of a valve, including manipulations and controls during the treatment and the catheters used, excluding the dilation catheter(s) and pharmaceutical and contrast products, maximum per operating session	Aortic arch / Aorta, thoracic descending	Repair (plasty)	Percutaneous transluminal	589201a	percutaneous endovascular aortic valve or congenital malformation of the thoracic without graft, percutaneous transluminal	
		Aortic valve	Implantation	Percutaneous transluminal	589201b	Aortic valve implantation, percutaneous transluminal [TAVI]	
		Mitral valve	Repair (plasty)	Percutaneous transluminal	589201c	Mitral valve plasty by trans septal puncture, percutaneous transluminal	
		Pulmonary valve / tricuspid valve	Repair (plasty)	Percutaneous transluminal	589201d	Pulmonary or tricuspid valve plasty, percutaneous transluminal	
		Aortic valve/mitral valve	Repair (closing)	Percutaneous	589201e	Paravalvular leakage closure, percutaneous	

Table 6.3. *An example of the pre-validator expert's contribution to the standardization of an ATMC*

NSS ATMC V1-3						
NSS ATMC V1-1		ICHI MAPPING				
Hospit modified code	Formulation	Target	Action	Means	ICHI Code	ICHI formulation
589201a	percutaneous endovascular aortic valve or congenital malformation of the thoracic without graft, percutaneous transluminal	Aortic valve or Aortic arch	Dilatation	Percutaneous transluminal	HDE.LG.AF or HIK.LG.AF	Percutaneous transluminal balloon dilatation of aortic valve or Percutaneous dilatation of aortic arch
589201b	Aortic valve implantation, percutaneous transluminal [TAVI]	Aortic valve	Implantation of internal device	Percutaneous transluminal	HDE.DN.AF	Percutaneous transluminal aortic valve replacement
589201c	Mitral valve plasty by trans septal puncture, percutaneous transluminal	Mitral valve	Dilatation	Percutaneous transluminal	HDF.LG.AF	Percutaneous dilatation of mitral valve
589201d	Pulmonary or tricuspid valve plasty, percutaneous transluminal	Pulmonary valve or Tricuspid valve	Dilatation	Percutaneous transluminal	HDG.LG.AF or HDH.LG.AF	Percutaneous transluminal dilatation of pulmonary valve or Percutaneous transluminal dilatation of tricuspid valve
589201e	Paravalvular leakage closure, percutaneous	Adaptation requested from WHO FIC				

Table 6.4. *Example of matching with ICHI*

It should be noted that ICHI is still in the development phase[9] and that this NPS ATMC V2 – ICHI matching is provisional.

For technical reasons, the codes identifying the procedures of the Belgian national nomenclature cannot exceed seven digits and must be numeric. ICHI codes and their extensions are not limited by these parameters. Therefore, the ICHI code cannot be substituted for the NPS code. Unlike the ICHI code whose triaxial logic is located within its codification, the NPS code does not contain any signification, which means that it does not allow for selective sorting. The latter can however be achieved from the three axes structuring the wording of the NPS ATMC V1. The matching table will enable the transmission, to international organizations (WHO, OECD, etc.) of the nature and volume of medical services provided in Belgium since each NPS ATMC V1 code corresponds to an ICHI code (within certain limits, see section 6.4.2).

6.2.4. *Provisional classification of new terms (NPS ATMC V1-3')*

The current NPS V0 nomenclature is a set of codes and formulations grouped by article, created and subdivided according to different circumstances. Most often, the articles cover more or less well- identified specialties, however, certain articles are "catch-alls" (Art.3, Art.11, Art.34, etc.). A total of 336 similar wordings with different codes are found in several articles.

A meaningful classification of medical procedures must be constructed on a rational basis. For example, an unambiguous formulation corresponds to a single code (bijectivity), the architecture of the classification must be hierarchical according to a uniform plan allowing easy navigation among the different subdivisions, etc.

The organization of the French *Classification Commune des Actes Médicaux* (i.e. Common Classification of Medical Procedures) or CCAM has been the subject of in-depth reflection by the ATIH[10] and Cnam[11] teams. The result is a model based on consistency. Rather than "reinventing the wheel", DESULB obtained permission from CCAM designers to use their classification system. Each term of the new nomenclature is complemented by a classification from the CCAM index (Table 6.5.).

---

9 An announcement by the WHO stating that ICHI is officially operational and exploitable is expected in October 2021.

10 *Agence technique de l'information sur l'hospitalisation* (i.e. Technical Agency for Information on Hospitalization).

11 *Caisse nationale d'assurance maladie* (i.e. National Health Insurance Fund).

N	NSS ATMC V1-3' Formulation	classification index
589201a	percutaneous endovascular aortic valve or congenital malformation of the thoracic without graft, percutaneous transluminal	04.02.02.01
589201b	Aortic valve implantation, percutaneous transluminal [TAVI]	04.02.02.07
589201c	Mitral valve plasty by trans septal puncture, percutaneous transluminal	04.02.02.01
589201d	Pulmonary or tricuspid valve plasty, percutaneous transluminal	04.02.02.01
589201e	Paravalvular leakage closure, percutaneous	04.02.02.07

CIRCULATORY SYSTEM
04.01 DIAGNOSTIC PROCEDURES ON THE CIRCULATORY SYSTEM
04.02 THERAPEUTIC PROCEDURES ON THE HEART AND ITS VESSELS
04.02.02 Therapeutic procedures on the heart valves
04.02.02.01 Dilation of the orifices of the heart
04.02.02.02 Orifice commissurotomy [Valvulotomy] or valvectomy
04.02.02.03 Cardiac annuloplasty and valvuloplasty [valvuloplasty]
04.02.02.04 Heart valve replacement
04.02.02.05 Reconstruction of fibrous rings of the heart
04.02.02.06 Reconstruction of the aortic pathway
04.02.02.07 Other procedures on the orifices of the heart

Table 6.5. *Each standardized act has a classification index*

To familiarize physicians with this new classification, adopted by INAMI as per the proposal of DESULB, the NPS ATMC V1-3 files are reclassified under this hierarchical presentation (NPS ATMC V1-3'). At this stage, the system is not based on a common inter-specialty classification but instead on a classification of the procedures of each specialty according to a common hierarchical classification model.

6.2.5. *INAMI administrative work*

At the end of the 18th week after the start of each of the six planned cycles, the result of the first four stages is sent to the INAMI, which is responsible for the translation from French into Dutch[12] and for the composition and coordination of the expert groups who will participate in the official medical validation.

6.2.6. *Validation of proposals by expert groups (NPS ATMC V1-4)*

During the 25th week of the cycle, the files adapted and translated by INAMI are sent to the experts.

The experts have four weeks to make their comments. These proposals must be sent in a structured form imposed by INAMI. Each proposal for any modification of the NPS ATMC V1-3 that has been sent to them must be written in a precise manner.

For instance, in the example shown in Table 6.6, the experts considered it useful to further subdivide the formulation. The NPS ATMC V1-3 file presented to them had subdivided the single procedure of NPS V0 (percutaneous endovascular aortic valve surgery, a congenital malformation of the aorta, of the pulmonary valve, of the mitral valve, of the tricuspid valve or fulguration of a valve, including manipulations and controls during the treatment and the catheters used, excluding dilation catheter(s) and pharmaceutical and contrast products, maximum per operating session) into five procedures. According to the experts, 16 formulations are needed to correctly describe these different procedures.

12 Belgium has two official national languages, as well as German for the small German-speaking community (a German translation is envisaged before the nomenclature is used for pricing purposes, in order to meet European regulatory provisions).

Hospit modified code	Target	Action	Means	NPS ATMC V1-3 wording
589201a	Aortic arch / Aorta, thoracic descending	Repair (plasty)	Percutaneous transluminal	percutaneous endovascular aortic valve or congenital malformation of the thoracic without graft, percutaneous transluminal
589201b	Aortic valve	Implantation	Percutaneous transluminal (femoral)	Implantation of an aortic valve, by femoral approach (TAVI).
589201p	Aortic valve	Implantation	Percutaneous transluminal (carotid)	Implantation of an aortic valve, by carotid approach (TAVI).
589201q	Aortic valve	Implantation	Percutaneous transluminal (direct aortic)	Aortic valve implantation, by direct aortic approach (TAVI).
589201r	Aortic valve	Implantation	Percutaneous transluminal (trans-apical)	Trans-apical aortic valve implantation (TAVI).
589201c	Mitral valve	Repair (plasty)	Percutaneous transluminal	Balloon mitral valve implantation, by endovascular approach and via trans-septal puncture
589201s	Mitral valve	Repair (plasty)	Percutaneous transluminal	Mitral valve implantation with clips, endovascular approach and trans-septal puncture
589201t	Mitral valve	Repair (plasty)	Percutaneous transluminal	Mitral valve implantation by ring implantation, endovascular approach and trans-septal puncture
589201u	Mitral valve	Implantation	Percutaneous transluminal (femoral	Mitral valve implantation via femoral artery approach
589201v	Mitral valve	Implantation	Percutaneous transluminal (trans-apical)	Mitral valve implantation via trans-apical approach
589201d	Pulmonary valve / tricuspid valve	Repair (plasty)	Percutaneous transluminal	Balloon implantation of the tricuspid or pulmonary valve via an endovascular approach
589201w	Tricuspid valve	Repair (plasty)	Percutaneous transluminal	Mitral valve implantation with clips, endovascular approach and trans-septal puncture
589201x	Tricuspid valve	Repair (plasty)	Percutaneous transluminal	Mitral valve implantation by ring implantation, endovascular approach and trans-septal puncture
589201y	Pulmonary valve / tricuspid valve	Implantation	Percutaneous transluminal (femoral)	Implantation of a pulmonary or tricuspid valve, by femoral approach
589201z	Pulmonary valve / tricuspid valve	Implantation	Percutaneous transluminal (trans-apical)	Trans-apical pulmonary or tricuspid valve implantation
589201e	Aortic valve/mitral valve	Repair (closing)	Percutaneous transluminal	Closure of a paravalvular leak, by endovascular approach

Table 6.6. *An example of modifications given by a group of experts for the proposed standardization work. For a color version of this table, see www.iste.co.uk/chaabane/healthcare.zip*

INAMI receives the expert proposals, which will be analyzed by a joint INAMI-DESULB team during the following two weeks.

The 31st and 32nd weeks should be devoted to meetings to discuss with the delegates from each expert group the observations and proposals of their group.

At the end of these meetings, a few weeks are scheduled to integrate the results of the validations and to make the desirable adjustments (NPS ATMC V1-4).

The entire process takes about 8 months for each batch of 450 procedures of the old NPS V0 nomenclature, on the understanding that there is overlap of successive cycles (e.g. the processing for Steps 1 through 4 of the second set of procedures will take place while Step 5 of the first batch of procedures is ongoing).

6.3. Results

6.3.1. *Planning*

1. Steps 1 to 4

The schedule for the first four stages was perfectly respected: 16 months after the beginning of the work, 1,698 ATMCs of the NPS V0 nomenclature were structured, standardized, pre-validated, matched and classified. This leaves only 975 to be processed. DESULB still has eight months to complete this task.

2. Step 5

INAMI follows the rhythm foreseen for the distribution of the restructured benefit tables to the expert groups who must validate this work (the 25th week of each cycle). For each group of experts (about 20 experts per specialty), a meeting to present and comment on the methodology followed and to assess the experts' initial observations was organized during the 30th week of each cycle. However, the processing of the experts' proposals is behind schedule.

6.3.2. *A summary of the modifications between NPS V0 and NSS V1-3*

Table 6.7 attempts to quantify the process that transforms the preparatory standardization work carried out by the DESULB team (NPS ATMC V1-2) into a standardized medical nomenclature that is sufficiently refined for it to be criticized by the groups of validating experts that will be convened by INAMI (made up of 20 standardized specialties and numbering 30 in total).

	ENT	Cardiac surgery	thoracic surgery	Pneumology	Cardiology	Urology	Abdominal surgery	OB-GYN	Gastroenterology	Plastic surgery	Vascular surgery	Stomatology	Ophtalmology	Dermatology	Hematology	Nephrology	Physiotherapy	Neurology	Neurosurgery	Spine surgery	Total
NSS V0	189	43	41	37	64	152	191	157	84	119	81	138	121	41	17	11	24	23	59	154	1.746
Steps 1 to 4: Analysis + Pre-structuring + Matching + Pre-validation																					
unique standardized labels	164	27	21	27	45	91	84	118	77	114	60	123	95	40	15	8	22	21	53	121	1.326
subdivisions	65	48	84	25	55	197	295	104	15	10	57	35	69	3	7	11	4	4	13	66	1.167
technical deletions	-33	-7	-18	-10	-16	-16	-38	-46	-12	-8	-10	-16	-34	-5	0	-3	-5	-8	-4	-2	-291
technical additions	6	6	34	6	6	34	127	12	9	9	4	18	7	1	0	0	2	9	3	0	293
obsolete deletions	4	3	1	3	2	13	12	4	0	6	7	1	4	1	0	0	4	0	6	1	72
new	1	0	0	0	3	3	7	10	5	0	0	2	15	2	3	5	0	5	0	0	61
NSS V1-3	202	74	121	48	90	306	468	188	89	125	111	160	137	39	22	16	23	26	65	185	2.495

Table 6.7. *A summary of the pre-standardization and pre-validation work. For a color version of this table, see www.iste.co.uk/chaabane/healthcare.zip*

The number at the top of the column indicates the number of codes in the current NPS V0 nomenclature that will need to be standardized. This number is higher than the one presented in Table 6.1 because it was decided, to avoid any frustration, that ATMCs performed in a proportion of more than 20% of the national total by one specialty will be presented to the experts of this specialty even if they are mostly performed by another specialty (e.g. the standardization of a procedure is thus successively validated by otolaryngologists, stomatologists and plastic surgeons, it being understood that a consensus must be found in order to arrive at one unique description).

Depending on the discipline, a greater or lesser number of ATMCs will have to be subdivided to meet the triaxial logic and to achieve a sufficient degree of precision when it comes to calculating rates. In the example of abdominal surgery, shown in the eighth column of Table 6.7, 107 of the 191 original procedures had to be subdivided and result in 295 procedures. The remaining 84 ATMCs have not been subdivided but the formulation has been modified, to a lesser or greater extent, to comply with the writing rules of the methodology.

As a result of standardization, procedures are duplicated or, to simplify the nomenclature, modifiers are added to a procedure thereby rendering other procedures unnecessary. For example, the following three terms "*examen échographique de la grossesse*" (i.e. ultrasound examination of pregnancy), "*examen échographique en cas de grossesse multiple*" (i.e. ultrasound examination in the event of multiple pregnancy) or "*examen échographique en cas de malformation congénitale grave*" (i.e. ultrasound examination in the event of severe congenital malformation) could be transformed into a single term "*examen échographique de la grossesse*" (i.e. ultrasound examination of pregnancy) covered by two modifiers ("*en cas de grossesse multiple*", i.e. "in the event of multiple pregnancy"; "*en cas de malformation congénitale grave*", i.e. "in the event of a serious congenital malformation"). The "duplicate" formulations or those which have become redundant due to modifiers will be the subject of a so-called "technical" deletion to differentiate them from the proposed deletions when a formulation is obsolete or no longer recommended according to good medical practice recommendations.

During the pre-validation work, it was noted that certain procedures are performed routinely but do not appear in the nomenclature and are the subject of assimilations to other existing procedures. The reform is an opportunity to update this by creating the corresponding formulation. Strictly speaking, these are not new procedures. They are technical additions, as opposed to innovations whose introduction is requested ("news"). The decision to admit these new medical techniques for reimbursement must follow a specific procedure.

To better reflect the work carried out during the steps leading to the standardization of formulations, we will distinguish between minor and major modifications.

a) Minor modifications are those which concern the formulations for which NPS V0 already implicitly contains the three structural axes, and which only require slight modifications to the syntax.

b) Major modifications are those concerning the wordings that are subdivided or deleted, the additions of services and the non-subdivided wordings that require major modifications to the structuring axes or syntax.

Overall, for the 20 disciplines concerned, 4% of the NPS ATMC V0 terms have been kept the same. The standardization work is made up of about 30% in minor changes and 66% in major changes. By comparison with the current nomenclature, the standardized and pre-validated nomenclature (ATMC) shows an increase of 43% in procedures. Of course, significant variations are observed depending on the discipline.

6.3.3. *Validation of proposals by experts (NPS ATMC V1-5)*

The expert groups of the different medical specialties, established by INAMI, received, on the dates specified in the schedules, tables of standardized medical documents translated into the two main national languages and proposals for classification on a uniform model. The expert groups from 13 specialties were brought together by INAMI within the prescribed deadlines. They had the opportunity to ask questions and express their opinions on the proposed restructurings. They were given precise directives indicating how they should send their observations, their proposals for modification and the introduction of new procedures. Halfway through Phase 1, eight of the 13 specialties whose procedures have been standardized had communicated their opinions. Section 6.4.4 provides an assessment of the nature of this validation work.

6.4. Discussion

As specified in section 6.1.4, this study is essentially descriptive. It is intended to pass on experience to those who face a similar challenge. The discussion will list the problems that still have to be solved to arrive at a common descriptive classification (section 6.4.1). This section will also provide some additional data concerning: the evaluation on the quality of the standardization work (section 6.4.2), the means mobilized to accomplish this work (section 6.4.3), the choice and participation of expert groups (section 6.4.4). Finally, it will be necessary to consider the implementation of a common descriptive classification of ATMCs (section 6.4.5).

6.4.1. *From the standardization of medical procedures to a common descriptive classification*

1) In section 6.2.4, we have only considered provisional classifications for the formulations of the new NPS ATMC V1 nomenclature. The relationship between the classification of procedures of the French CCAM and that of procedures for future Belgian nomenclature was described. It was specified that the partial classifications carried out are limited to classifying the procedures of each specialty studied, according to the scheme adopted for the CCAM. At this stage, it is only a question of intra-disciplinary classifications according to a uniform scheme. The objective is educational: to familiarize Belgian physicians with the classification style that will be adopted for future Belgian classification.

Phase 1 will not conclude in September 2021 when the last batch of formulations in the NPS V0 nomenclature has been standardized, sent to INAMI and validated by the experts. This first phase will only be completed once all the standardized formulations are integrated into a common descriptive classification (CC ATMC V1)[13].

Based on the initial provisional common classifications created from the already standardized ATMCs, it is estimated that it will take several months to arrive at this point (Table 6.8).

Several additional works will still be necessary: (a) the integration of the experts' proposals will require numerous arbitrations, which will only be possible once the procedures of all the specialties have been standardized; (b) working by specialty creates duplicates, which will have to disappear according to the principle of bijectivity; (c) the pairing with ICHI should be fully verified and updated once the official version of this classification is announced by WHO; finally, (d) it will be necessary to update, complete and describe the methodological guide necessary for the subsequent maintenance of the common classification; and (e) ensure that the final product (CC ATMC V1) does indeed comply with the requirements of this guide.

13 And once the consultation work with clinical biology, pathology and radiotherapy is completed.

INAMI Code & Libellé NSS V1		RIZIV Code & Omschrijving NGV V1		ICHI Code & Descriptor	
05.03 ACTES THÉRAPEUTIQUES SUR LE S		**05.03 THERAPEUTISCHE VERSTREKK**		**05.03 THERAPEUTIC INTERVENTIONS ON THE HAEMATOPOIETIC AN**	
05.03.01 Actes thérapeutiques sur la		**05.03.01 Therpeutische verstrek**		**05.03.01 Therapeutic interventions on the spleen**	
05.03.01.01 Évacuation de collecti		**05.03.01.01 Evacuatie van sple**		**05.03.01.01 Drainage of spleen collection**	
242653a	drainage d'abcès ou de kyste	242653a	drainage van miltabces o	DJA.JB.AA	Drainage of spleen
242653b	drainage d'abcès ou de kyste	242653b	drainage van miltabces o	DJA.JB.AB	Laparoscopic drainage of spleen
05.03.01.02 Splénectomie		**05.03.01.02 Splenectomie**		**05.03.01.02 Splenectomy**	
242XX3a	splénectomie partielle, par a	242XX3a	partiële splenectomie, via	DJA.JJ.AA	Partial splenectomy
242XX3b	splénectomie partielle, par c	242XX3b	partiële splenectomie, via	DJA.JJ.AB	Laparoscopic partial splenectomy
242631a	splénectomie totale, par abor	242631a	totale splenectomie, via o	DJA.JK.AA	Total splenectomy
242631b	splénectomie totale, par coel	242631b	totale splenectomie, via e	DJA.JK.AB	Laparoscopic total splenectomy
05.03.01.03 Autres actes thérape		**05.03.01.03 Andere therapeu**		**05.03.01.03 Other therapeutic interventions on the spleen**	
242771a	splénorraphie, par abord ouv	242771a	splenorafie, via open ing	DJA.MK.AA	Repair of spleen
242771b	splénorraphie, par coeliosco	242771b	splenorafie, via endosco	DJA.MK.AB	Laparoscopic repair of spleen
08 APPAREIL URINAIRE ET GÉNITAL		**08 URINAIR EN GENITAAL STELSEL**		**08 GENITOURINARY SYSTEM**	
08.01 ACTES DIAGNOSTIQUES SUR L'AP		**08.01 DIAGNOSTISCHE VERSTREKKI**		**08.01 DIAGNOSTIC INTERVENTIONS ON THE GENITOURINARY SYST**	
08.01.02 Échographie de l'appareil u		**08.01.02 Echografie van het urin**		**08.01.02 Ultrasound of the genitourinary system**	
469291	échographie du petit bassin,	469291	echografie van het kleine	NMZ.BA.BJ	Ultrasound of female pelvis, NOS
08.01.07 Ponction, biopsie et prélèv		**08.01.07 Punctie, biopsie en pre**		**08.01.07 Biopsy of the genitourinary system**	
08.01.07.04 Ponction, biopsie et p		**08.01.07.04 Punctie, biopsie e**		**08.01.07.04 Biopsy of the female genital system**	
149612	frottis cervico-vaginal, effect	149612	cervicovaginaal uitstrijk	(NMF.AH.AC&XXNMH)&01	Cervical papanicolaou smear, vagina
149634	frottis cervico-vaginal effectu	149634	cervicovaginaal uitstrijk	(NMF.AH.AC&XXNMH)&02	Cervical papanicolaou smear [follow-
432110	biopsie du col de l'utérus, pa	432110	biopsie van de baarmoe	NMF.AD.AC	Cervical biopsy
432132	biopsie de l'endomètre, par v	432132	biopsie van het endometr	NME.AD.AC	Transvaginal biopsy of uterus

Table 6.8. *The common classification will allow for the transition from French into Dutch and into English. For a color version of this table, see www.iste.co.uk/chaabane/healthcare.zip*

2) The reader will wonder why the initiators for the structural reform of the Belgian nomenclature did not simply adopt the whole of the CCAM instead of limiting themselves to its own method of classification.

In Europe, as in the United States or Australia, one of the main uses of nomenclatures is linked to financing, in particular when fee-for-service (FFS) financing is one of the dominant methods for paying physicians (which is largely the case in Belgium). From this perspective, nomenclature is a sensitive subject on which the attention of physicians, hospital managers, insurers and the State is focused. In addition, attached to this type of fee-based nomenclature is a set of descriptions that are supplemented by tariffs and many application rules. Belgian physicians were ready to accept a modernization of their nomenclature based on the principles that underpin modern classifications. Simply transposing another classification would have meant making a political choice which, given the country's federal structure, would have required endless discussions on the comparative merits and limits of different national classifications.

Finally, the CCAM, like other nomenclatures, is not exempt from criticisms (excessive granularity, the creation of adverse effects) imposing a revision that has become essential according to the task force appointed by the French government to propose health reforms ("*Ma santé 2022*", i.e. My Health 2022).

6.4.2. *Evaluate the quality for the standardization of medical procedures*

We knew that our current NSS V0 nomenclature was obsolete and that modernizing the terms was a necessary measure. We imagine that the process described above contributes to significantly improving the quality of the future NSS ATMC V1, though this is only a subjective assessment.

To measure the value of the work carried out more objectively, we undertook a comparison with the WHO ICHI classification with the assumption that the latter could serve as a reference. This study was presented in summary form at the WHO annual classifications meeting (Leclercq 2020). In summary, a random sample of 130 medical procedures was selected from the 1,333 already standardized medical procedures (10 procedures for each of the 13 medical specialties being addressed during the first 12 months of the study). The level of equivalence between ICHI and the Belgian nomenclature was estimated before standardization (NPS V0 – ICHI) and after standardization (NPS V1 – ICHI) according to a method recommended by a Swedish team (Almborg *et al.* 2017). Three codification specialists, familiar with the old (NSS V0) and the new Belgian nomenclature (NPS V1), as well as ICHI, determined the level of equivalence for the 130 procedures in the sample. While the

NPS V0 – ICHI equivalence level was only 46.5% and the NPS V0 was more accurate than ICHI in 14.7% of cases, for the NPS V1 – ICHI comparison, these indicators are improving considerably (equivalence: 63.6%; superior accuracy of NPS V1: 24.1%). For these comparisons, only the ICHI "stem" code was used.

6.4.3. *An estimate of the resources mobilized to arrive at a common descriptive classification*

The standardization and pre-validation of half of the NPS V0 formulations (1.333 ATMC) corresponding to the medical activity of 13 medical and surgical specialties, as well as the matching to ICHI of 1.333 standardized terms required approximately 1,675 hours of preparatory work. The medical pre-validation mobilized 140 hours of physicians' time and a further 360 hours worktime by the DESULB team.

To these estimates, we should also add the training time of the DESULB team by the physician expert in medical classification; other preparatory work such as the drafting of a provisional standardization manual, the study of ICHI and the participation in the validation work of this international classification; the work carried out within the INAMI and the work carried out by expert groups.

6.4.4. *Participation of medical experts*

The descriptive phase for the reform of the Belgian nomenclature of medical benefits mobilized three categories of medical experts.

1) As indicated in section 6.2.2, a medical classification expert trained the DESULB team for several months on the constraints imposed by rigorous standardization. During this period, the expert also matched the new terms of the NPS ATMC V1 with the CCAM, a subject on which he is well acquainted. In this way, we were reviving previous studies that compared the NPS V0 with the CCAM (Pirson *et al.* 2004; Leclercq and Pirson 2005). By systematically matching the labels of the NPS ATMC V1 with the CCAM, we wanted to explore the possibility of using the statistical information of the CCAM for the benefit of the pricing studies provided for in Phases 2 and 3 of the Reform Plan for Belgian nomenclature. This work was the subject of an article recently submitted for publication (Leclercq *et al.* 2020a).

2) The role of the experts in charge of medical pre-validation was explained in section 6.2.2. They are physicians chosen for their reputation within their discipline. They work closely with the DESULB team, systematically reviewing

pre-standardized terminology, answering questions, specifying structural elements (topography, action, means) and suggesting minor or major modifications to the work being presented to them. It is at once both very dense and rewarding teamwork over the course of which DESULB regularly recaps on the objectives and rules to be respected.

3) The choice of expert groups from different specialties responsible for validating the standardization work is the responsibility of INAMI, which has opted for a very broad selection. INAMI has indeed solicited universities, medical societies, professional and trade union associations, and insurance organizations, asking them to suggest physicians interested in the subjects dealt with. The experts therefore represent a wide variety of entities (physicians from private and public hospitals, university and non-university institutions, Dutch-speaking and French-speaking physicians, physicians from insurance organizations and trade union physicians).

It is not always easy to make this range of "experts" understand that it is a question of the development of a precise and updated descriptive classification, and not a tariff classification, which will be the subject of subsequent steps. The expert groups meet among themselves without receiving any "coaching" from INAMI or DESULB. Even if the examination of the tables offered to them by INAMI (NPS ATMC V1-3) must follow an imposed methodology, the feedback is not of a similar quality. Some documents correspond perfectly to the work requested, while other proposals are poorly presented without respecting the INAMI guidelines. Some experts want to anticipate the pricing phases and think what they find in the multiplication of formulations or modifiers is a technique to promote their discipline. Others exhaust themselves in internal discussions, split into sub-working groups and are slow to return the results of their labors.

After a broad opening to all the actors in the field, INAMI hopes that each expert group will propose one or two coordinators with whom the analysis of the validation work can be carried out methodically. If we want to achieve a concrete result for Phase 1 within a reasonable timeframe (standardized term integrated into a definitive common descriptive classification), a mixed INAMI-DESULB team will have to restore coherence in this accumulation of disparate proposals.

6.4.5. *The implementation of common descriptive classification (CC ATMC V1)*

The reform plan includes three phases: the development of a common descriptive classification is a prerequisite followed by two studies, one intended for the calculation of professional fees and the other for the calculation of operating costs related to the performance of medical procedures. The first phase has been estimated to take three years, while the second phase, for which preparatory work has already been carried out (Leclercq and Pirson 2018), could take anywhere between three and five years. The design of Phases 2 and 3 is hardly compatible with the phased introduction of the new tariffs. There will therefore be a considerable gap between the end of Phase 1 and the implementation of the new tariffs.

Theoretically, three options are possible: (1) the CC ATMC V1 is "stored" for three to five years while waiting for new tariffs, (2) the NPS V0 is used concurrently for tariff purposes and the CC ATMC V1 for statistical and epidemiological purposes, and (3) from 2022, the CC ATMC V1 is implemented as both an instrument for pricing and as a method of recording data for statistical and epidemiological purposes.

1) This option seems unlikely. INAMI realizes that it will be difficult to keep CC ATMC V1 up to date for several years if potential users are not aware of its existence. In addition, having announced a structural reform in 2019, after mobilizing a significant budget and several dozen medical experts, to announce that it will be necessary to wait until 2025 before seeing the first changes does not appear to be a very rational approach.

2) For Phases 2 and 3, quantified data on recorded medical activity recorded based on the CC ATMC V1 will be needed. This could be achieved by good sampling and dual recording: NPS V0 for pricing and NPS ATMC V1 for statistical data. Recording the same activity using two coding systems is very burdensome for institutions, which will require financial means to meet their additional costs. It is also a source of potential errors and is hard to justify unless it is for a limited period (6 to 12 months). After a few months, we will therefore find ourselves in a situation comparable to scenario 1 outlined above.

3) The third option is probably the only realistic one. In summary, in 2022 the CC ATMC V1 would be declared "fit for service" and "provisionally" priced. To achieve this result, it is necessary to transpose the tariffs and rules of the NPS V0 to the CC ATMC V1 by declaring that it is a transitional phase while Phases 2 and 3 are studied. These transpositions are complex but not impossible. DESULB has studied them and presented them to INAMI. The decision will have to be made in a timely manner as it will take several months of preparation to transform the descriptive CC ATMC V1 into a provisional pricing CC ATMC V1. Among the other questions to be resolved, there will be a need to upgrade software because the codification system of the NPS V1 involves numerous technical adaptations.

6.5. Conclusion

The development or modernization of a descriptive nomenclature of medical procedures can be prepared by trained teams (specialized nurses, medical technologists). This approach saves time for physicians. A small, highly specialized team can ensure compliance with standardization rules, a steady pace of progress and provide valuable support in arbitrating among the multiple "expert" proposals. In addition, this team will be able to contribute very actively to many additional tasks such as the completion of Phase 1 or the preparation of a transitional pricing phase.

Medical expertise is obviously essential, but it is also necessary to regulate the discussions to ensure that the basic principles are respected and that financial ulterior motives are removed from this essentially descriptive phase.

Having a modern classification of medical procedures instead of obsolete nomenclature is a matter of satisfaction, even more legitimate as the efforts to achieve it are considerable. However, in the absence of a strategy proposing a way to benefit from such an instrument, discouragement, frustration and criticism are to be expected. Since there is no way back, and a wait-and-see attitude is hardly sustainable, the only option is to opt for the interim fee-based CC ATMC V1 and do everything possible to make it work.

6.6. References

Almborg, A.-H., Vikdal, M., Berg, L. (2017). Method and rules when mapping various classifications of procedures with ICHI. Poster, WHO–Family of International Classifications Network Annual Meeting, Mexico.

CCAM (2001). Une nouvelle nomenclature : pourquoi ? Comment ? Quand ? *CNAMTS*, 1–6.

Conney, A.H., Lou, Y.R., Xie, J.G., Osawa, T., Newmark, H.L., Liu, Y., Chang, R.L., Huang, M.T. (1997). Some perspectives on dietary inhibition of carcinogenesis: Studies with curcumin and tea. *Proceedings of the Society for Experimental Biology and Medicine*, 216(2), 234–245.

Devillé, L., Dierckx, H., Kesteloot, K., Laurent, A., Leclercq, P., Vleugels, A. (1993). Réajustement des honoraires médicaux, herijking van de medische honoraria. Final report, Ministère Fédéral des Affaires Sociales et Algemeen Syndikaat van Genneskundigen van België, 1–42.

Dizdaroglu, M., Jaruga, P., Rodriguez, H. (2003). Oxidative damage to DNA: Mechanisms of product formation and measurement by mass spectrometric techniques. In *Critical Reviews of Oxidative Stress and Aging*, Cutler, R.G., Boucher, D. (eds). World Scientific Publishing, Singapore.

Duroudier, J.-P. (2016). *Thermodynamics*. ISTE Press, London, and Elsevier, Oxford.

Flipo, F. (2018). *The Coming Authoritarian Ecology*. ISTE Ltd, London and John Wiley & Sons, New York.

Leclercq, P. and Pirson, M. (2005). Comparaison de nomenclatures d'actes médicaux : impacts de l'utilisation des nomenclature belge (INAMI) et française (CCAM) sur la rémunération d'une équipe chirurgicale. *Journal d'économie médicale*, (1), 37–55.

Leclercq, P. and Pirson, M. (2018). Réforme du financement des hôpitaux. La problématique des honoraires médicaux (Frais de fonctionnement et travail médical). Definitive Report, January, 1–460.

Leclercq, P. and Pirson, M. (2019). Réforme structurelle de la nomenclature des soins de santé INAMI. *Plan Cadre*, 1–49.

Leclercq, P., Devillé, L., Dierickx, M., Sylin, M., Bériot, I. (1996). Développement d'une méthodologie de réajustement des honoraires médicaux en Belgique. *Phase II : étude de consensus sur les critères permettant d'objectiver les poids relatifs des différentes activités*, Definitive Report, 1–160.

Leclercq, P., Pirson, M., Azzi, D., Bardiaux, S., Van den Bulcke, J. (2019). Actualisation de la méthodologie de standardisation des libellés de procédures médicales. *Intermediary report to the l'INAMI*, 1–22.

Leclercq, P., Melin, N., Van den Bulcke, J., Bardiaux, S., Azzi, D., Pirson, M. (2020a). La réforme de la nomenclature belge des procédures médicales pourrait-ellle profiter de l'expérience de la Classification commune des actes médicaux ? *Revue d'épidémiologie et de santé publique*, (68-S1), 30-31.

Leclercq, P., Pirson, M., Azzi, D., Bardiaux, S., Van den Bulcke, J. (2020b). Reform of the Belgian health nomenclature (progress report and matching with ICHI). *Virtual meeting, WHO–Family of International Classifications Network Annual Meeting*.

Ma santé (2022). Rapport de la Task Force "Réforme du Financement du système de santé" [Online]. Available at: https://solidarites-sante.gouv.fr/IMG/pdf/dicom_rapport_final_vdef_2901.pdf.

Pirson, M., Patris, A., Leclercq, P., Bodin, J.-P. (2004). Financement des blocs opératoires en France et en Belgique. *Journal d'Economie Médicale*, 4, 177–187.

7

Digital Toolkit for the Ergonomic Evaluation of Workstations

7.1. Introduction

Thanks to the introduction of information technologies, scientific methods and the mass of available data, health and healthcare centers will soon be able to prevent, anticipate, monitor and follow the evolution of public health so as to better intervene at the right time with the right tools.

In this context, ergonomics will increasingly occupy a place within these health and healthcare centers. We can cite a few examples of workstations that require special attention at the ergonomic level: people who lift and move loads, those who install and handle patients, those in charge of placing meal trays on trolleys for distribution in patient rooms, etc.

Ergonomics offers solutions to eliminate injury to human health or well-being in the workplace. In other words, ergonomics adapts professional activity to human characteristics.

With a proportion of almost 2% of GDP in Europe, work-related musculoskeletal disorders (MSDs) account for the majority of occupational health injuries, well ahead of work-related accidents. The term MSD refers to a set of painful disorders involving muscles, tendons and nerves, by and large related to frequent and repetitive activities.

Moreover, ergonomic workstations are a legal obligation for the employer. In general, we observe that the implementation of ergonomic measures can significantly reduce absenteeism. Therefore, preventative solutions in this area provide value as they contribute to financial saving by reducing the absence rate.

Chapter written by Valentin ROCHAT and Antoine HAYEK.

ProcSim, which is very active in the health sector and whose mission is to help its customers make the right decision in terms of flow and process in the digital transformation of their company, places importance on the well-being of people in their professional environment. Specialized in flow management and process optimization of dynamic systems through 3D modeling, simulation, analysis, optimization, prediction and visualization, ProcSim also offers its services and digital tools in the field of ergonomics.

7.2. ProcSim and ergonomics

7.2.1. *Origin*

Through numerous collaborations with clients in the industrial, health and transport sectors, we have found that improvement efforts are very often focused on the technical performance of machines, equipment and processes, but often the (perhaps) most important aspect is forgotten: the human element. For example, on a production line, we could have the most efficient machine in the world, but if the work place occupied by the operator is not ergonomic, the overall technical performance of the line will never reach the value theoretically foreseen at the design stage.

It was after this realization that we decided, with the help of the *Centre suisse d'électronique et de microtechnique*, or the CSEM (i.e. the Swiss Center for Electronics and Microtechnology), to develop the first digital toolkit for the ergonomic evaluation of workstations.

It is important to note that this tool is intended to complement the current observation methods carried out by ergonomists and not to replace them. It offers the customer ergonomic results and scores, in a digital, automated and objective manner.

7.2.2. *Our product*

Our digital toolkit therefore makes it possible to assess the ergonomics of a workstation. This takes into account the human being within the systems analysis. This tool can be used in existing or even future workplaces. For these and for all workstations with problematic access, the use of a 3D simulation model as well as standard equipment for virtual reality (mask, controllers) is necessary.

The goal is to offer companies an innovative solution in the form of a "ready-to-use" kit, consisting of body sensors and a software including 3D simulation and virtual reality packages.

The CSEM has therefore developed sensors and tags that are placed at certain strategic points on the body, dependent on the task being performed. The measurements are not intrusive for staff and last a maximum of 15 to 20 minutes. They can be repeated several times according to the different sizes of people and take into account movements, angles, working time, the nature of the terrain and surfaces. Once the parameters are saved, these are processed and modeled by the 3D simulation software from ProcSim.

Digitization makes it possible to simulate a large number of profiles very quickly, which makes it possible to prescribe, through virtual reality, the best layout appropriate for a given industry, workplace and/or person.

This solution is based on ergonomic rating standards that meet the requirements of current standards, such as EN 1005. According to the standard being used, the ergonomic risk index of a workstation is then categorized into four sections:

- work posture;
- application of force;
- load transport;
- repetitive upper body movements.

Other factors could also be taken into account such as the environment (noise, temperature, vibration), stress, etc.

7.2.3. *Examples of applications in different sectors*

We have already been able to test our tool in the industrial sector thanks to a collaboration with Nestlé. In fact, as part of a test phase in the Cailler chocolate factory in Switzerland, we were able to put our technology to the test on a substantial production line in Broc, France. This test allowed us to realize all the benefits and enormous potential of this innovation.

As far as the health sector is concerned, we have already been able to apply our toolkit to two institutions. First, with a large pharmaceutical company in order to assess a visual inspection station, where the operator performs quality checks on vials. And second, with a university hospital center as part of the construction of a new hospital logistics platform.

For this last project, our toolkit was used to achieve two goals. The first was to train operators in their new working environment, using the virtual reality tool. The second was to study and evaluate the ergonomics of these new workplaces.

The outcomes of this project were very positive because, in addition to the ergonomic analysis and its results, the information resulting from the virtual reality models brought real added value to the operators. Having already been aware of the changes that would take place in their workstations, they were able to adapt more easily with fewer misconceptions during the transition phase.

7.2.4. *Benefits and value addition*

As mentioned above, the goal of ProcSim in integrating ergonomics into its approach is to put people back at the center. To this end, we have set ourselves clear objectives. We are committed to improving comfort and well-being; preventing musculoskeletal disorders in order to limit absenteeism as well as increasing employee productivity at their workstations.

Our tool helps improve existing workstations and design better workstations for the future. In addition, it is important to mention that the ergonomic dimension is fully integrated in the analysis of the technical performance of the position within its environment.

In terms of added value, through this digital assessment, we deliver quantifiable results and ergonomic scores based on standards such as “RULA” and “EAWS”.

From the customer’s point of view, our solution provides the following advantages:

– the standardization of the ergonomic assessment of their establishments in order to be able to create benchmark references between their different sites or positions;

– the quantified improvement of workplaces based on relevant performance indicators;

– the use of a digital and objective approach as a complement to the work of ergonomists;

– the identification of potential non-human workstations that could eventually be replaced by robots.

7.3. Ergonomic assessment process

7.3.1. *Data collection*

We start by collecting the data that interests us through IMU sensors that can be placed on:

– the head;

– the torso;

– the upper arms;

– the forearms;

– the hips;

– the hands.

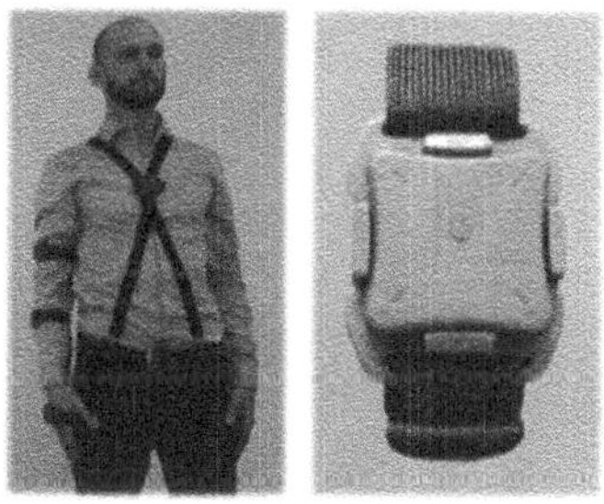

It is important to note that the calibration of IMU sensors is based on the exact movement of the body part where it is being tested.

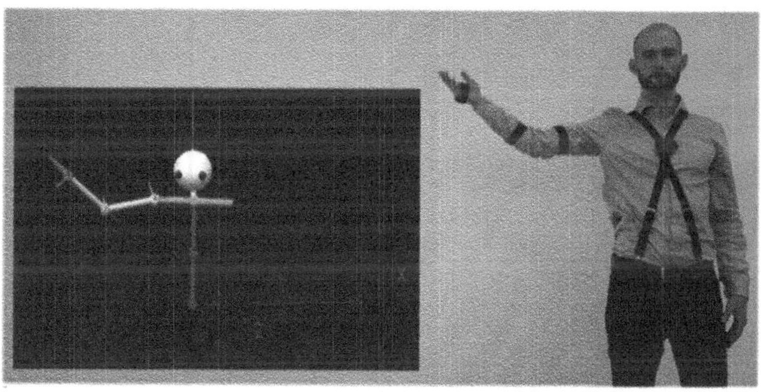

Figure 7.1. *Data collection. For a color version of this figure, see www.iste.co.uk/chaabane/healthcare.zip*

7.3.2. *Data analysis*

Next, we use ergonomic standards such as "EAWS" and "RULA" to analyze the data in the best possible way. The simple purpose of choosing to integrate these international ergonomic standards is to achieve an optimal level of relevance when analyzing the data collected.

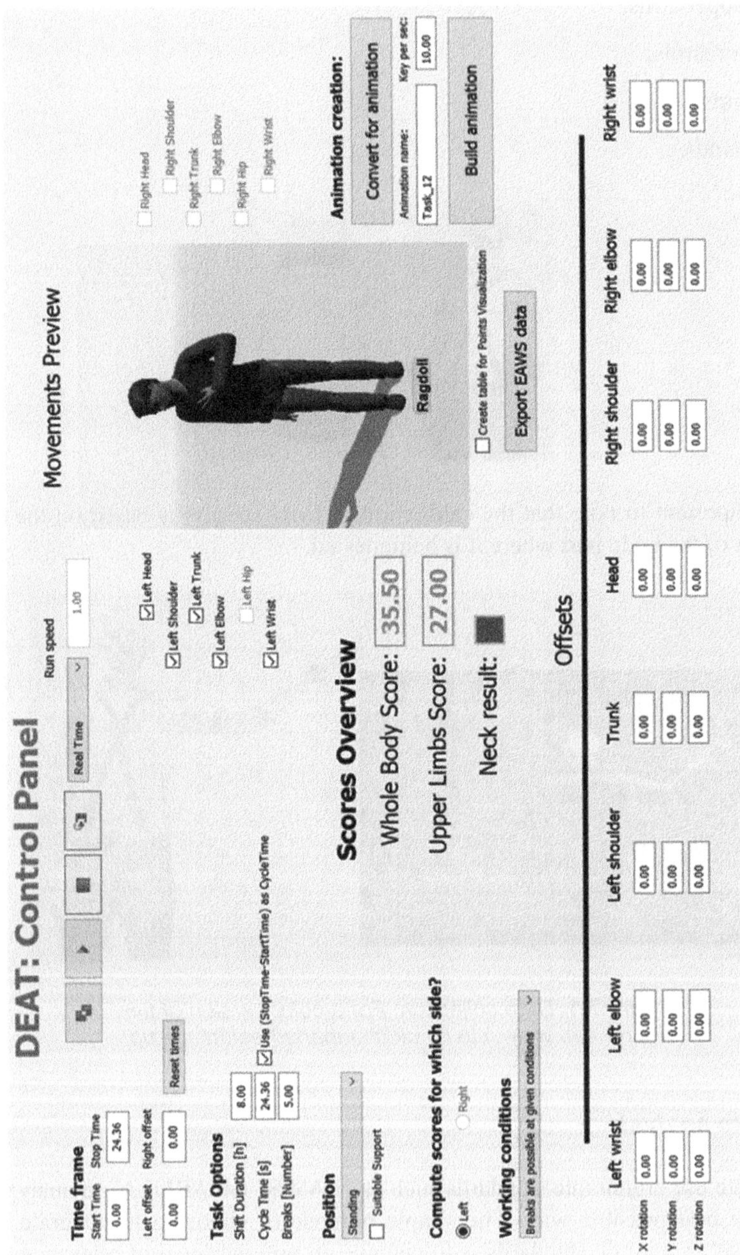

Figure 7.2. *Analysis of collected data. For a color version of this figure, see www.iste.co.uk/chaabane/healthcare.zip*

7.3.3. *Workstation modeling*

When the data collection and analysis is done, we model the entire system around the workstation and integrate the operator and their 3D animation.

The ergonomics of the workplace will have an impact on the technical performance of the entire system. Hence, it is important to consider it as an integral part of our approach.

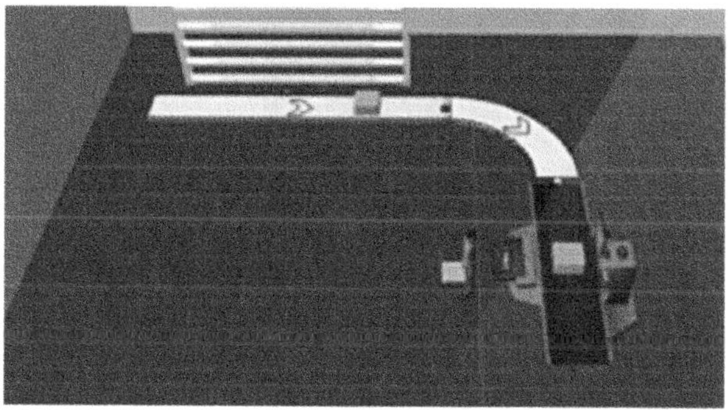

Figure 7.3. *Workstation modeling. For a color version of this figure, see www.iste.co.uk/chaabane/healthcare.zip*

7.3.4. *Virtual reality testing of possible activities*

This phase can be very useful in improving the scope of the analysis. The use of virtual reality is essential in three situations:

– challenging the design of a future workstation;

– testing improvements on existing workstations;

– studying workstations that are difficult to access.

In addition, this tool can be used to represent operators' animations directly in their work environment.

7.3.5. *Improvement proposals and recommendations*

Once the data collection and analysis process are complete, we offer our clients areas for improvement as well as relevant recommendations according to the industry and the reality on the ground.

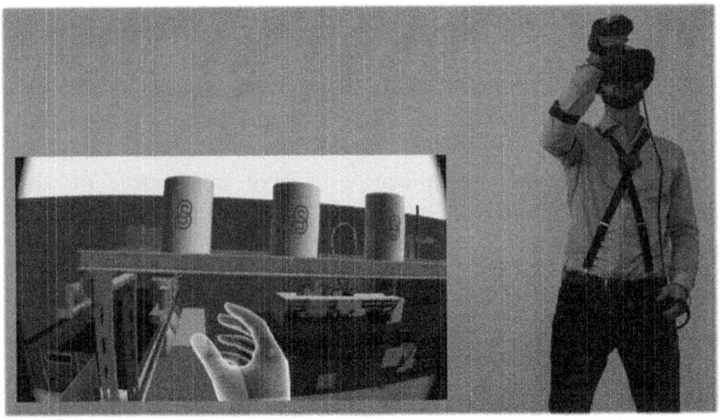

Figure 7.4. *Virtual reality tests. For a color version of this figure, see www.iste.co.uk/chaabane/healthcare.zip*

7.4. Conclusion

Our real added value in the field of ergonomics is our ability to consider the workstation as a whole and integrate it directly into 3D simulation models of the entire environment.

Along with our expertise in flow management and process optimization, we assist our clients to make the right decision while considering the well-being of their employees to carry out their professional activities.

Our goal is to complement the ergonomist's expertise through observation. Our digital tool provides a quantified and objective analysis based on recognized standards. It also allows for a benchmark reference between different yet similar workstations, on different sites. Note that the introduction of cameras could constitute future development of our tool.

To conclude in line with the theme of GISEH 2020 (which promotes agile management in health and healthcare establishments to be integrated into their environments whilst remaining efficient), it is important to remember that the health and well-being of the human being in such an environment, like that of a hospital, is a key standpoint. As a result, our ergonomic toolkit allows people to be put in the place they should be occupying, that is, at the center of concerns, all the while improving the overall performance of health and healthcare establishments.

7.5. References

ACGIH (2001). Association Advancing Occupational and Environmental Health [Online]. Available at: https://www.acgih.org/.

Bruere, S. (2017). Histoire de l'ergonomie [Online]. Available at: https://managersante.com/2017/06/12/ histoire-de-lergonomie/.

Buchholz, B., Paquet, V., Punnett, L., Lee, D., Moir, S. (1996). PATH: A work sampling-based approach to ergonomic job analysis for construction and other non-repetitive work. *Applied Ergonomics*, 27(3), 177–187 [Online]. Available at: http://www.sciencedirect.com/science/article/pii/ 000368709500078X.

Colombini, D., Occhipinti, E., Álvarez Casado, E. (2013). OCRA: Revised OCRA checklist [Online]. Available at: http://www.ergonomiesite.be/documenten/repetitief/Revised-OCRA-Checklist-Book.Pdf.

CSEM (2021). CSEM [Online]. Available at: https://www.csem.ch/home.

Delalande-Danet, V., Desarmenien, A., Incorvaïa, A.M., Letheux, C., Leviel, C., Viossat, M. (2015). *Les troubles musculo-squelettiques*. CISME, Paris.

e-RSE (2019). Ergonomic : définition, exemples et domaines d'application [Online]. Available at: https://e-rse.net/ergonomie-definition--exemple-application/.

EAWS (N/A). EAWS: Design the way to work [Online]. Available at: http://www.eaws.it/.

FlexSim (2021). Simulation software for manufacturing, material handling, healthcare, etc. [Online]. Available at: https://www.flexsim.com/.

GISEH (2020). Site internet du GISEH 2020 [Online]. Available at: https://www.uphf.fr/evenements/giseh2020.

Grimmault, Y. (2018). Ergonomic assessment of repetitive tasks in Virtual Reality. Technical report, EPFL, Lausanne.

GS1 (2018). 18e GS1 Forum Suisse de Logistique [Online]. Available at: https://www.gs1.ch/fr/home/offre/%C3%A9v%C3%A9nements/2018/18e-gs1-forum-suisse-de-logistique.

Gueniat, P. (2017). Ergonomic evaluation using movement measurement technics and 3D simulation. Technical report, EPFL, Lausanne.

Life Performance Research (2019). Life Performance Research [Online]. Available at: https://lp-research.com/.

Martinet, P. (2018). Workplace ergonomics 3D analysis module using IMU technology and virtual reality. Technical report, EPFL, Lausanne.

Meunier, P. (2010). Le combat des ergonomes suisses pour mieux faire reconnaître leur profession. *Le Temps* [Online]. Available at: https://www.letemps.ch/economie/combat-ergonomes-suisses-mieux-faire-reconnaitre-profession.

Procsim (N/A). Procsim: Make the right decision [Online]. Available at: https://procsim.ch/.

RAMP (2017). Risk management assessment tool for manual handling proactively [Online]. Available at: https://www.ramp.proj.kth.se/ramp-1.730128.

Tar-Ching, A.W., Gardiner, K., Harrington, J.M. (2006). *Occupational Health*, 5th edition. Wiley-Blackwell, Malden, MA.

8

Simulation on an RFID Interactive Tabletop with Tangible Objects of Future Working Conditions: Prospects for Implementation in the Hospital Sector

8.1. Introduction

In an increasingly competitive world in which technologies evolve rapidly, companies, as is the case for most organizations in general, must adapt, reorganize and transform. It is therefore essential that methods are put in place so that employees, whatever their profile, can, in particular, be trained so as to better take ownership of new working conditions. Different types of methods centered on the human factor are possible, for example, around paper/cardboard prop simulators or virtual reality (Pastré 2005; Van Belleghem 2012, 2018).

The method proposed in this chapter is based on a set of advances in the field of human–computer interaction, particularly with regard to tangible interaction (Ishii and Ullmer 1997; Shaer and Hornecker 2010), as well as from the perspective of serious gaming and gamification (Abt 1970; Adams 2006; Ma *et al.* 2011; Alvarez and Djaouti 2012; Alvarez *et al.* 2017), to move towards the proposal of a simulator on an interactive tabletop with tangible objects.

This simulator is in line with the work carried out on the TangiSense Interactive tabletop that has been equipped with RFID technology (Kubicki *et al.* 2013, 2015; Lebrun *et al.* 2014, 2015; Havrez *et al.* 2016; Bouabid *et al.* 2018; Lepreux *et al.* 2018; Merrad *et al.* 2019). Such a simulation approach aims to encourage the

Chapter written by Yoann LEBRUN, Nicolas VISPI, Sophie LEPREUX, Sondès CHAABANE and Christophe KOLSKI.

involvement of employees in collective situations, in relation to a set of scenarios, using a fun approach, promoting training and employees taking ownership of future working conditions.

This chapter begins with the state of the art on the simulation of working conditions, with the objectives of training and employees taking ownership. It then describes the global principle of simulation through the use of an interactive tabletop, as proposed in this chapter. Next, the proposed simulation tool is presented and illustrated via its various functionalities. The chapter ends with a set of perspectives offered by this interactive tool, relative to the hospital sector.

8.2. State-of-the-art on the simulation of future working conditions

Yesterday's transformation projects, whether technical, architectural or organizational, have forged today's working conditions. In fact, today's projects will define the working conditions of tomorrow. By this logic, being able to project ourselves in a secure manner, in a new environment, in a new organization, has always been of particular interest (Maline 1994), for both designers and prevention specialists; and this, regardless of the type of simulation under consideration: retrospective, reflective, projective or prospective (Bobillier Chaumon *et al.* 2018).

Initially based on traditional supports (2D plans, volumetric models), we are witnessing a democratization of simulation tools, including 3D modeling and virtual reality (through head-mounted displays or as an immersive space), which have great potential: quality of immersion, precision of data, coupling and data collection (postural, eye-tracking) facilitating decision-making. However, the experience feedback shows a measured use, mainly by large companies due to the human (modeling, preparation, animation) and financial costs of these technologies, but also because of its techno-dependent aspect.

For the most part, envisaged within the framework of architectural projects, the development of an organizational simulation (Van Belleghem 2012; Daniellou *et al.* 2014) that mobilizes classic props, such as paper, models and other physical objects, has made it possible to extend the conceivable use of the simulation of future working conditions to other objects, such as management or skills development. This has also made it possible to envisage broader deployment prospects, in particular those pertaining to very-small and medium-sized enterprises (VSEs/SMEs).

The healthcare sector is no stranger in using simulations. The "SimuSanté" centers of the CHU d'Amiens (i.e. Amiens University Hospital), or even "Presage" of the CHU de Lille (i.e. Lille University Hospital), illustrate the use of simulation well as an educational means in initial and continual training, to train the best healthcare practices, or specific practices or situations, but remains focused on healthcare. In another example, Cheyrouze and Barthe (2018) use scripting tools in their work to identify the strategies put in place for organizations working 12-hour shifts. While identifying the strategies is necessary, it is not necessarily transformative. Ultimately, simulation in the hospital sector remains concentrated on care or identifying action strategies. In both cases, it seems that the quality of care and quality of working conditions are disconnected.

8.3. Proposal for a simulator on an interactive tabletop

The principle of a simulator, developed on an interactive tabletop associated with inert and active tangible objects, is proposed. It aims to support activity simulations by following a participatory and interactive approach, according to innovative simulation principles. The objective of the simulator is to offer an interactive, pleasant support, allowing employees to take ownership of new work situation(s). Indeed, with this simulator, several people can simultaneously collaborate around the tabletop, using a set of objects that have been qualified as tangible (see Figure 8.1). Activities can also involve other actors at other times, so as to gradually integrate changes and assess the effect of certain solutions. The simulation of the activity (work or use) aims to help individuals (agents, users) to project themselves into the activities that will make up their role in this environment. It therefore makes it possible to simulate potential future working conditions, as well as the management or development of skills and competencies.

To do this, the exchange between project stakeholders (operators, designers, project manager, decision-makers, partners, etc.) is facilitated by the simulator. In addition, the computerization of the sequences allows the modification of design choices until the simulated activity is considered acceptable, by the participants, to meet the challenges of the project (working or usage conditions, quality requirements, the service provided to the user, etc.). In this regard, the simulator must make it possible to represent the prescribed scenarios (space, equipment, etc.) and its possible evolutions; it must also allow the various actors to operate or suggest modifications to the prescribed scenarios shown on the tabletop.

User interaction with the interactive tabletop through tangible objects (such as avatars) aims to facilitate ownership in the workplace (Van Belleghem 2012). Other objects used can take different forms in order to represent the spaces to be fitted out (office, reception, resuscitation room, etc.) and the equipment to be positioned (computer, automaton, chair, stretcher, etc.) in a playful and transitional way, and simulate the activity of the user(s) via the avatar objects mentioned above.

Figure 8.1 shows a cycle of use for the interactive tabletop in three stages (as suggested by Van Belleghem (2012)), in which the simulation has diverse and complementary interests, as several cycles may be necessary depending on the project.

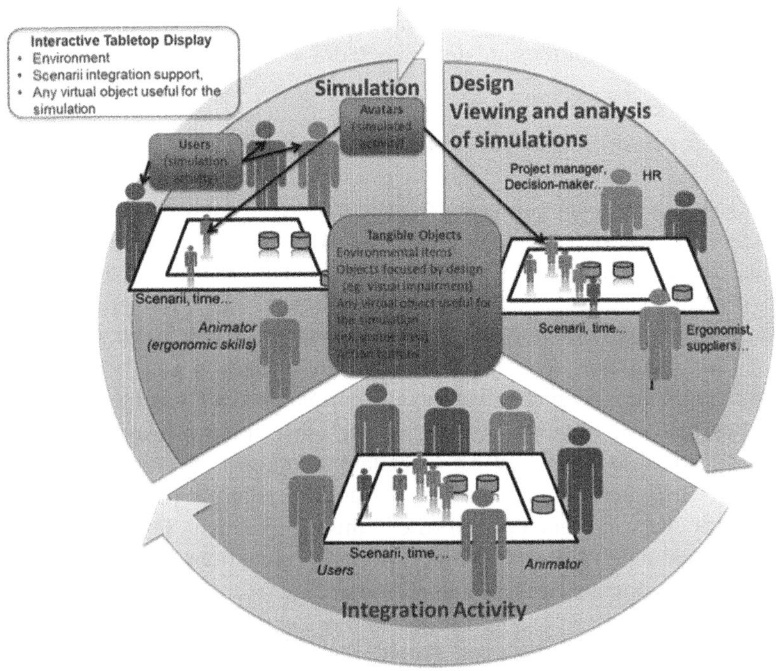

Figure 8.1. *The three stages of the activity simulation process of an interactive tabletop and tangible objects. For a color version of this figure, see www.iste.co.uk/chaabane/healthcare.zip*

Step (1), called "Simulation", allows users to utilize the simulator to project themselves into the new activity or activites. It is also possible to utilize it to project the user into current and future situations in order to make comparisons.

The so-called "Design" Step (2) uses the previously recorded trace logs, as part of one or more simulation sessions. Decision-makers can thereby become aware of potential repercussions for users from the various options that may have been proposed during the "Simulation" step.

Finally, Step (3), called "Integration", allows the user to review the choice(s) made. It thus allows the user to envisage their future way of working, in their new environment.

8.4. Development of a first version of a simulator on an interactive tabletop

The proposed simulator was developed on the TangiSense interactive tabletop (http://www.rfidees.com). TangiSense is equipped with RFID technology, allowing for the manipulation of tangible and traceable objects (Kubicki *et al.* 2009). The tabletop is equipped with a full HD screen, allowing the user to be more immersed in the world of simulated reality.

The simulator on an interactive tabletop allows for exchange between actors of a project and the modification of design choices until the simulated activity is considered acceptable, by the participants, to meet the challenges of the project (working or usage conditions, quality requirements, service provided to the user, etc.). Consequently, this first version of the simulator meets several objectives:

– It allows for the representation and modification of prescribed elements in the form of scenarios (keeping trace logs of changes in prescribed scenarios).

– It allows for the collective modification of prescribed scenarios (everyone can authorize themselves to move the elements on the interactive tabletop, the designer is associated with the discussions).

– It allows for the simulation of an activity with avatars. The avatars (figurines) allow actors of the simulation to transpose themselves by *playing* the scenarios, that is, imagining themselves in a situation by moving the object, embodying the future situation in order to really simulate it and not be limited to a prescribed scenario that does not take user experience into account, that is, facilitating the move from the third person perspective (i.e. "*one*") to the first person perspective (i.e. "*I*") (Van Belleghem 2012);

– It makes provisions for digital interactions.

– It allows for the visualization of processes and flows. This is to allow for the representation of avatar movements during the simulation. This representation indicates both the position of the avatars in space and the length of time the avatar remains in one place.

– It allows for a scenario to be replayed by modifying the typical parameters (e.g. task durations, work environment arrangements, number of operators involved in the activities).

– It assists in data analysis through statistical analysis. Indeed, once the simulation, graphs and/or tables are generated, it makes it possible to quickly and easily take a stance on the movements of the avatar. For designers and decision-makers, this means, for example, studying alert points (bottlenecks, oversaturation, etc.).

Figure 8.2 shows the simulator using the interactive tabletop onto which different objects are placed. This makes it possible to combine both the tangible (via objects) and the virtual (via the interactive tabletop screen) objects. The objects represent the avatars (characters) and the various arrangements (tables, pallets, beds, etc.). When objects move, they indicate the distance traveled thanks to the scale integrated into the map. They also leave trace logs of their passage.

Potential users involved in the apparatus are:

– *facilitators/ergonomists*: these users have first conducted a study of the existing activity, if it exists, and have prepared the simulation (e.g. actors/users, experts (see below) and/or non-experts). These are the users who prepared the scenarios and typical situations;

– *investment experts*: present during the simulation or participating remotely, the architects, developers, builders/suppliers, as well as internal or external project owners;

– *non-experts*: employees, actors in a simulation of their activity, with different levels of qualification;

– *decision-makers*: these are business or department heads, elected officials or even volunteer managers;

– *employee representatives*: employee representatives, *Comité d'hygiène, de sécurité et des conditions de travail* (i.e. Health, Safety and Working Conditions Committee) or CHSCT;

– *end users*: patients, students, etc.

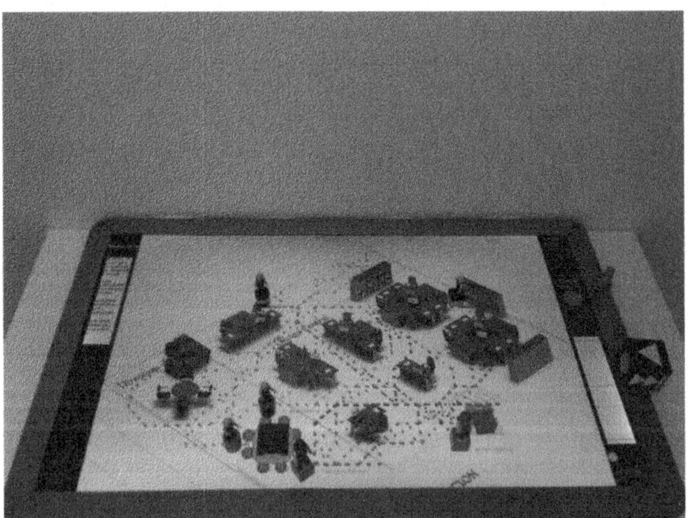

Figure 8.2. *Example of a simulation on an interactive tabletop. For a color version of this figure, see www.iste.co.uk/chaabane/healthcare.zip*

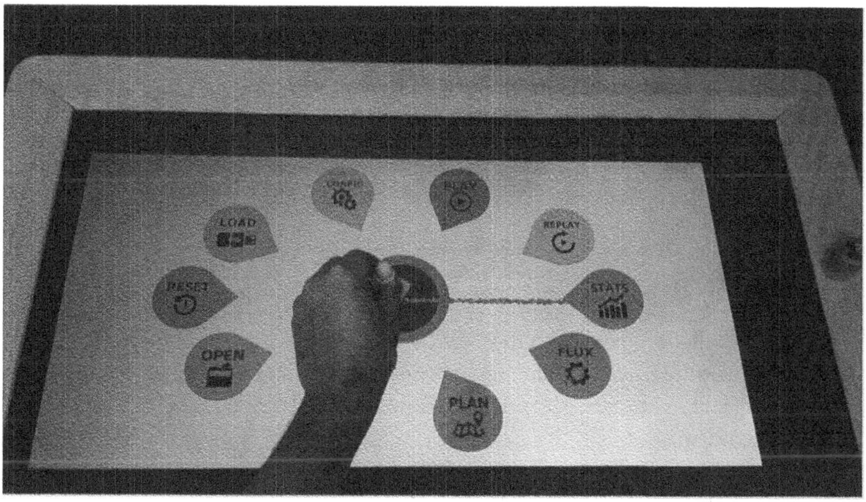

Figure 8.3. *Drag and drop stats menu selection. For a color version of this figure, see www.iste.co.uk/chaabane/healthcare.zip*

Figure 8.3 shows the simulator menu and its different functionalities. This menu is made up of the following modes:

– CONFIG: allows the user to configure objects equipped with an RFID tag so that they are recognized in the simulation tool. This mode is made up of two parts:

- Definition of facilities: it is with this functionality that we place any object equipped with an RFID tag to associate it with an image. In addition to being associated with an image, this object can have functionalities within the simulation. It can have the role of tracking this image (in the form of a shadow) or the role of replicating this image as many times as you want (in the form of a stamp). Indeed, it is judicious to define an object buffer type if the image needs to be represented many times within the simulation. This avoids defining a large number of tangible objects for the same image.

- Definition of the characters: it is with this functionality that we place any object equipped with an RFID tag to associate it with a given character. We consider two types of characters/avatars. Internal avatars (e.g. company employees) and external avatars (e.g. delivery person, someone external to the company). After placing an object in one of the zones, it is also possible to assign it a color. This color will be used in the simulation (e.g. to draw the movements of the avatar). This color can be used to distinguish the roles of the characters (e.g. blue for a production manager, green for a worker, etc.).

Therefore, it is possible to potentially place an infinite number of RFID tags, as well as upload a very large number of images. Indeed, in order to make the application as autonomous as possible, it is possible to add new images into the configuration library (see the LOAD module).

– PLAY: allows the user to play a simulation according to a plan and a prescribed scenario.

– REPLAY: allows the user to replay a simulation.

– STATS: allows the user to display the statistics of a simulation over time.

– FLOWS: allows the user to define flows and insert them within the simulation. It is about generating digital elements in order to realistically simulate the movement of users, objects, vehicles, etc. These flows are integrated and adapted to the different scenarios.

– PLAN: allows the user to select a plan (or an image) and load it into the simulation or define/modify its scale.

– SAVE: allows the user to save the simulation so as to replay it later, or to export it.

– OPEN: opens a simulation that has been saved.

– RESET: allows the user to reset the simulation tool by deleting all plans, backup folders, images, instructions, etc.

– LOAD: allows the user to import graphic elements (images, plans) into the simulation tool, as well as scenarios in the form of a spreadsheet file. The system analyzes the USB keys connected to the computer, browses all of the images and makes them available to the user. When images are loaded, they then automatically appear in the Image Library; in addition, it allows the user to export backups (from USB storage media).

In order to access this menu, the user must use a specific object. This "menu" object is instantiated in the simulator and cannot be modified by other users. After placing the object to access the menu, the user must first place it on one of the modes and then move it to the center of the menu into the "validate here" area. This principle is used throughout the different modes to express choices or validations.

Furthermore, within the simulator, the object has its own definition. This means that if the user defines an object's functionality for the first time, the next time the simulation is started it will be automatically recognized. The key advantage of this solution is that it eliminates the need to define the behavior of tags/objects for future simulations, since their definition has already been saved. This saves time and avoids having to define all of the objects each and every time the system is started.

8.5. Application opportunities in the healthcare industry

Simulation has been extensively used in the healthcare system for the purposes of training focused on care or identifying action strategies. The purpose of these simulators was focused on the quality of care. A lot of the other work on simulation has been oriented towards problems with pilot programs or hospital logistics (Kadri *et al.* 2014). This work focused on the organizational aspects, but the involvement of nursing staff was mainly in the phases of identifying needs and validating the results. Unfortunately, these simulations were not concerned with working conditions, interprofessional interactions or the setting up of new organizations involving nursing staff throughout the simulation phases. It is for these reasons that our simulator could find its place in the hospital world by promoting a better-informed response to organizational issues. We have thus identified three potential applications of the simulator.

The first opportunity addresses strained situations involving environments that are hectic and tiring for both caregivers and patients. We have worked on these strained situations in emergency departments, from the perspective of patient flow during epidemic periods (Kadri *et al.* 2014). Our results have shown that it is not enough to simply increase human or material resources; we need to rethink the way we manage flows and waiting rooms. This management system can effectively contribute to the reduction of these situations. The simulator could therefore be used in the context of improving working conditions in emergency services. This entails the involvement of caregivers in the design of a new organization that aims for better flow management. It is about rethinking their workspace and the entire environment, not just from the point of view of flow, but also from the point of view of the caregiving process. The advantage of a simulator not only allows caregivers to project themselves, but also to test, simulate and virtually experience situations ranging from a known and experienced epidemic (e.g. gastroenteritis, flu, etc.) to more complicated scenarios, and even crisis situations. We could also involve the patients themselves; for instance, when working with pediatric emergencies, where parents can think of different perspectives to given scenarios. The Covid-19 pandemic is a good example of a situation that has highlighted organizational and communication difficulties (Sang and Trimi 2021; Wang *et al.* 2021). The simulator could be used to allow health professionals to reproduce the choices made in reaction to the pandemic, in order to identify the dysfunctions of these choices and propose and test new organizations with the benefit of hindsight and more information.

The second opportunity concerns how health personnel take ownership of new technological advances, such as the installation of a new robotic cabinet in a central pharmacy department, assisting in the delivery of medication services for a hospital. This technological development could bring improvements in terms of logistics, medication management and error rate, but involves a reorganization of services, as pointed out by Cousein (2014) and Blanchard Petrini (2015). The simulator could allow users to participate in a simulation showcasing the introduction of these cabinets in the pharmacy, and the organizational impacts this entails. This would give them the opportunity to think about new organizations, test them and make suitable changes. They could thus test against extreme situations, as specified above, and calculate indicators related to the safety of the medication circuit.

The last opportunity relates to the concept of teamwork and the interprofessional context, which are very important aspects of the hospital environment. The interactive tabletop and the concept of *serious games* could facilitate the implementation of role-playing games and allow different health professionals to be involved in the collective resolution of problems and in the proposition of solutions. This will also identify mechanisms for interprofessional communication, which is one of the key elements of patient safety, as specified in the report by the Australian Council for Safety and Quality in Health Care (2005). In the same vein, the simulator could be used to test the cohesion of a healthcare team, set up coordination mechanisms and identify interaction problems around a serious game simulating the real functioning of the service concerned. In this regard, it should be remembered that the concepts of team, communication and interaction have been identified as being essential elements for the proper functioning of healthcare services (Dumas *et al.* 2016).

8.6. Conclusion and perspectives in the healthcare industry

The simulation and ownership of future working conditions leads to significant discussion in many areas. Interactive tabletops associated with tangible objects provide new solutions on this subject. One such solution has been presented within the framework of this chapter. By bringing together digital and analog technologies, the simulator presented in this publication allows for a wider deployment by reducing costs, and the intervention of an expert is not required. This has been observed within the framework of the simulator deployment since 2015 as a regional tool for the Hauts-de-France region: the Hauts-de-France *Association Régionale pour l'Amélioration de Conditions de Travail* (i.e. Regional Association for the Improvement of Working Conditions), or ARACT. The regional innovation and development agency have established collaborations within the regional system framework known as "Industrie du Futur" (i.e. Industry of the Future) and were able to implement simulations for future working conditions within various companies.

In the healthcare system, simulation has the exclusive objective of healthcare. The tool presented offers the possibility of an organizational simulation which reconciles organizational efficiency and quality healthcare. This seems all the more important in light of the Covid-19 pandemic, which has highlighted the organizational dysfunctions in the sector and their direct impact on healthcare quality.

Such an approach can be generalized to many other sectors of activity, particularly to Industry 4.0, which needs to rapidly change its processes and organizational methods (Vispi *et al.* 2020).

8.7. Acknowledgments

The authors of the chapter warmly thank Marie-Christine Lenain, who was involved in the initiation of the simulator. They also wish to thank Julian Alvarez, who spoke on the *Serious Game* aspects of the simulator, as well as Laurent Van Belleghem for his active participation in the *Integratic* seminars. They would also like to thank the Hauts-de-France Region, which supported the development of the simulator. Last but not least, this chapter is dedicated to their colleague and friend Professor Christian Tahon.

8.8. References

Abt, C. (1970). *Serious Game*. Viking Press, New York.

Adams, E. (2006). *Fundamentals of Game Design*. New Riders Pub, New York.

Alvarez, J. and Djaouti, D. (2012). *Serious Games: An Introduction*. Questions Théoriques, Limoges.

Alvarez, J., Plantec, J., Vermeulen, M., Kolski, C. (2017). RDU model dedicated to evaluate counsels for Serious Game projects. *Computers & Education*, 114, 38–56.

Australian Council for Safety and Quality in Health Care (2005). National patient safety education: Framework & bibliography. Document, Australian Council for Safety and Quality in Health Care, Canberra.

Blanchard Petrini, B. (2015). Sécurisation du circuit du médicament et automatisation des PUI : intérêts et pratiques. Thesis, Ecole des Hautes Etudes en Santé Publique, Rennes.

Bobillier Chaumon, M.-E., Rouat, J., Laneyrie, E., Cuvillier, B. (2018). De l'activité DE simulation à l'activité EN simulation : simuler pour stimuler. *Activités*, 15(1).

Bouabid, A., Lepreux, S., Kolski, C. (2019). Design and evaluation of distributed user interfaces between tangible tabletops. *Universal Access in the Information Society*, 18(4), 801–819.

Cheyrouze, M. and Barthe, B. (2018). Travail de nuit en 12 heures : un scénario de travail élaboré par les infirmiers dans un service de réanimation. *Activité*, 15(1).

Cousein, E. (2014). Rôle du pharmacien hospitalier dans la sécurisation et l'optimisation de la prise en charge médicamenteuse du sujet âgé. Clincal pharmacy PhD Thesis, Université de Lille 2, Lille.

Daniellou, F., Legal, S., Promé, M. (2014). Organisational simulation: Anticipating the ability of an organisation to cope with daily operations and incidents. In *11th International Symposium on Human Factors in Organizational Design and Management (ODAM)*, Broberg, O., Fallentin, N., Hasle, P., Jensen, P.L., Kabel, A., Larsen, M.E., Weller, T. (eds). Danmarks Tekniske Universitet, Copenhagen.

Dumas, M., Douguet, F., Fahmi, Y. (2016). Le bon fonctionnement des services de soins : ce qui fait équipe ? *RIMHE : Revue interdisciplinaire management, homme & entreprise*, 20(1), 45–67.

Havrez, C., Lepreux, S., Lebrun, Y., Haudegond, S., Ethuin, P., Kolski, C. (2016). A design model for tangible interaction: Case study in waste sorting. *IFAC/IFIP/IFORS/IEA Symposium on Analysis, Design and Evaluation of Human-Machine System*, Kyoto, 373–378.

Ishii, H. and Ullmer, B. (1997). Tangible bits: Towards seamless interfaces between people, bits and atoms. *CHI '97 Conference Proceedings*, ACM, Atlanta, GA, March 22–27.

Kadri, F., Chaabane, S., Tahon, C. (2014). A simulation-based decision support system to prevent and predict strain situations in emergency department systems. *Simulation Modelling Practice and Theory*, 41, 32–52.

Kubicki, S., Lepreux, S., Lebrun, Y., Dos Santos, P., Kolski, C., Caelen, J. (2009). New human-computer interactions using tangible objects: Application on a digital tabletop with RFID technology. In *Human-Computer Interaction, 13th International Conference, HCI International 2009, Proceedings, Part III (San Diego, July 19–24)*, Jacko, J.A., Stephanidis, C., Harris, D., Schmorrow, D.D., Grootjen, M., Karsh, B.-T., Shumaker, R., Zaphiris, P., Ozok, A.A., Duffy, V.G., Kurosu, M., Smith, M.J., Salvendy, G., Aykin, N., Estabrooke, I.V. (eds). LNCS, Springer-Verlag.

Kubicki, S., Lebrun, Y., Lepreux, S., Adam, E., Kolski, C., Mandiau, R. (2013). Simulation in contexts involving an interactive table and tangible objects. *Simulation Modelling Practice and Theory*, 31, 116–131.

Kubicki, S., Wolff, M., Lepreux, S., Kolski, C. (2015). RFID interactive tabletop application with tangible objects: Exploratory study to observe young children' behaviors. *Personal and Ubiquitous Computing*, 19(8), 1259–1274.

Lebrun, Y., Lepreux, S., Haudegond, S., Kolski, C., Mandiau, R. (2014). Management of distributed RFID surfaces: A cooking assistant for ambient computing in kitchen. *5th International Conference on Ambient Systems, Networks and Technologies, ANT-2014* (Hasselt, Belgium, June 2–5), Procedia Computer Science, Elsevier, Amsterdam.

Lebrun, Y., Adam, E., Mandiau, R., Kolski, C. (2015). A model for managing interactions between tangible and virtual agents on an RFID interactive tabletop: Case study in traffic simulation. *Journal of Computer and System Sciences*, 81, 585–598.

Lepreux, S., Alvarez, J., Havrez, C., Lebrun, Y., Ethuin, P., Kolski, C. (2018). Jeu sérieux pour le tri des déchets sur table interactive avec objets tangibles : mise en œuvre et évaluation. *Ergo'IA '18, Proceedings of the 16th Ergo'IA "Ergonomie et Informatique Avancée" Conference (3–5 October)*, ACM, Bidart.

Ma, M., Oikonomou, A., Jain, L.C. (2011). *Serious Games and Edutainment Applications*. Springer-Verlag, London.

Maline, J. (1994). *Simuler le travail. Une aide à la conduite de projet*. Editions de l'ANACT, Montrouge.

Merrad, W., Habib, L., Héloir, A., Kolski, C., Krüger, A. (2019). Tangible tabletops and dual reality for crisis management: Case study with mobile robots and dynamic tangible objects. *ANT 2019, The 10th International Conference on Ambient Systems, Networks and Technologies* (April 29 – May 2), ANT, Leuven.

Pastré, P. (2005). *Apprendre par la simulation – de l'analyse du travail aux apprentissages professionnels*. Octarès Editions, Toulouse.

Sang, M. and Trimi, S. (2021). Convergence innovation in the digital age and in the COVID-19 pandemic crisis. *Journal of Business Research*, 123, 14–22.

Shaer, O. and Hornecker, E. (2010). Tangible user interfaces: Past, present and future directions. *Foundations and Trends in Human-Computer Interaction*, 3(1), 1–138.

Van Belleghem, L. (2012). Simulation organisationnelle : innovation ergonomique pour innovation sociale. In *Innovation et travail : sens et valeurs du changement*, Dessaigne, M.-F., Pueyo, V., Béguin, P. (eds). Actes du 47ème Congrès de la SELF, 5–7 September, Lyon.

Van Belleghem, L. (2018). La simulation de l'activité en conception ergonomique : acquis et perspectives. *Activité*, 15(1).

Vispi, N., Lebrun, Y., Lepreux, S., Chaabane, S., Kolski, C. (2020). Simulation on RFID interactive tabletop of working conditions in industry 4.0. *SOHOMA 2020, 10th Workshop on Service Oriented, Holonic and Multi-Agent Manufacturing Systems for Industry of the Future*, October, Paris.

Wang, Y., Hao, H., Platt, L.S. (2021). Examining risk and crisis communications of government agencies and stakeholders during early-stages of COVID-19 on Twitter. *Computers in Human Behavior*, 114, 106568.

9

Robotic Geriatric Assistant: A Pilot Assessment in a Real-world Hospital

9.1. Introduction

In the context of an aging population, the assessment and monitoring of elderly patients contributes to the objectives of geriatric preventative care, namely to extend lifespan without disability and to preserve autonomy. Proposed by Dr. Marjory Warren as early as the 1930s (Matthews 1984), the comprehensive geriatric assessment (CGA) is a multidimensional and multidisciplinary diagnostic tool for the medical, psychosocial and functional (in)capacities of the elderly (Stuck *et al.* 1993). The CGA is considered the gold standard for frailty management (Turner *et al.* 2014; Nord *et al.* 2021). This health check is the basis for developing a coordinated and adequate care plan, promoting healthy aging. However, the proposal for this type of screening and follow-up is currently insufficient when compared with the growing elderly population: a large proportion of the frail elderly population is currently not being taken care of, or insufficiently.

The research hypothesis is that a robotic solution would improve efficiency in geriatric follow-up, thus allowing for the identification and follow-up of a greater number of elderly people. Since the comprehensive geriatric assessment is standardized, certain tests – in particular, where it concerns functional disabilities – can be automated and delegated to the robotic geriatric care assistant, making it possible to optimize clinicians' time on activities with high added value, such as drawing up the care plan. The result of three years of research, *Clara* is now an operational robot geriatric care assistant at the technology readiness level – TRL 8 level.

Chapter written by Dimitri VOILMY, Karine LAN HING TING, Ana IGLESIAS, Rebeca MARFIL, Juan Pedro BANDERA, Fernando FERNANDEZ and Quitterie DE ROLL.

For a color version of the figures in this chapter, see www.iste.co.uk/chaabane/healthcare.zip.

This chapter presents the pilot assessment which was carried out in real-life situations between May and July 2019, as part of a framework partnership agreement between the institutions that some of the authors are stationed at. In its review of the literature on social robot studies, one of the shortcomings noted by Broekens *et al.* (2009) concerns methodological failure: short-term experiments and only vague descriptions of the results. The analysis of the social acceptance of social robots in the domestic context (de Graaf *et al.* 2015) highlights the need for long-term studies. This would, according to the authors, mitigate against the novelty effect. Indeed, people's perceptions of robots, their behaviors and their experiences, are likely to change over time. It is in line with this recommendation from studies – those that are long-term, in real environments, with a sufficient number of users – alongside previous research by some of the authors (Lan Hing Ting *et al.* 2018), which motivates part of this geriatric assistant robot evaluation research presented in this chapter.

9.2. Geriatric assessment: from needs to the proposed solution

The geriatric assessment is usually performed every six months and involves both patients and their families. It includes three different types of activities: a clinical interview, a multidimensional assessment and a personalized care plan. First of all, the clinical interview allows the patient and their relatives to discuss the health problems of the elderly person with the doctor. Next, the multidimensional clinical tests are performed to assess the general condition of the patient. Finally, taking into account the data collected during the two previous phases, and the evolution of the patient since the last assessment, the geriatrician establishes a personalized care plan.

Some of these activities require the presence of clinical staff, but others, notably the multidimensional assessment, are standard tasks that lend themselves to automation and/or parallelization (for more details, see Lan Hing Ting *et al.* (2017) and Voilmy *et al.* (2017)). It is inconceivable to replace the human caregiver with the services of a robot. The use of this assistance robot must in no way replace any human presence, according to the robo-ethical principle (Nevejans 2017), applied from the earliest beginnings of this research. The research hypothesis examined, in particular during the evaluation described in this chapter, that the partial delegation of tasks to a medical assistance robot would allow clinicians to concentrate on activities with higher added value, such as the collaborative development of the appropriate care plan, in conjunction with the patient and their family. However, according to a second ethical principle, the patient needs to give prior consent for this robot assistant in geriatrics to take charge.

The comprehensive geriatric assessment differs from the standard medical assessment in three ways: (i) it focuses on older people with chronic conditions; (ii) it emphasizes functional status and quality of life; and (iii) it usually entails an interdisciplinary team, which requires the coordination of several professionals. This coordination is largely based on the sharing of patient data.

9.2.1. *Data management and the proposed robotic solution*

Data management is also part of the robotic solution described in this chapter. It combines a professional application, called CGAmed, and a robot geriatric assistant, called Clara, by the research team following participatory living lab workshops (see Figure 9.1 below). The CGAmed physician application allows the clinician to configure the tests to be performed. After that, the robot can autonomously perform the tests and save the results in the application database. Finally, the clinician will use the application again to review the results of the session, create a new care plan and develop patient follow-up (see the detailed presentation of the solution in works by Lan Hing Ting *et al.* (2017) and Voilmy *et al.* (2017), including the system architecture (Bandera *et al.* 2016, 2017b)). Conjointly, CGAmed and the Clara robot perform all the functions involved in the collection of geriatric data, as normally enacted by clinicians (described in Lan Hing Ting *et al.* (2018)): querying, collecting, extracting and sharing patient data, so that it can be interpreted by clinicians as part of the collaborative development of the care plan.

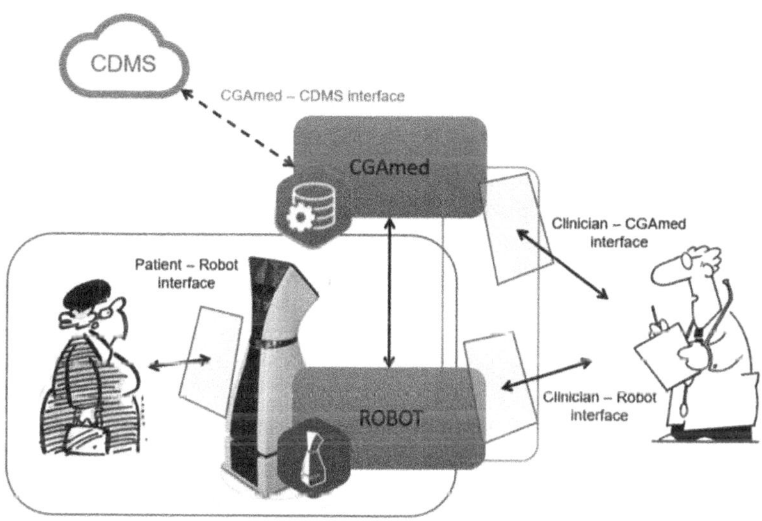

a)

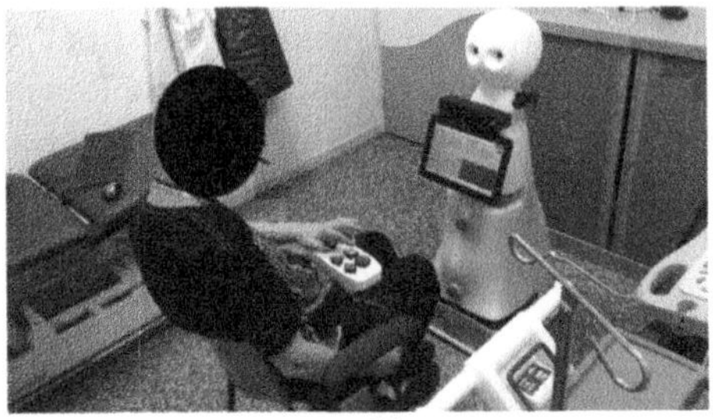

b)

Figure 9.1. *(a) Overview of the robotic system; and (b) a real patient interacting with Clara (right)*

This chapter deals more specifically with the interaction with the Clara robot, which amalgamates the characteristics of a mobile service robot. The medical use of this new type of assistive robotics for medical personnel is an entire topic in its own right and not detailed here. The main idea to keep in mind is that it appears to be a promising option, due to the robot's inherent proactivity, autonomy, adaptability and potential acceptability (Feil-Seifer and Mataric 2005). As a stand-alone robotic solution to support geriatric assessment, Clara will need to provide conditions of effective implementation regarding the collection of relevant data from the patient. During the geriatric tests, Clara collects, records and displays the responses, offering four possible modes of interaction: voice, touch screen, remote control buttons and motion detection.

During this pilot assessment, two tests were applied to the robot: the *Barthel* test (a functional test relating to the instrumental activities of daily life, which takes the form of a questionnaire) and the *Get up & Go* test (evaluating locomotion and the quality of balance, via an analysis carried out by the Kinect camera integrated into the robot). Indeed, the medical Clara robot assistant is able to deploy all the functionalities required by the questionnaires and motion-based tests – including natural language, face tracking and detection, and human motion capture.

9.2.2. *The Clara robotic geriatric assistant – research*

The Clara robot tested in this pilot assessment is a functional robot at the TRL8 level. The design of interfaces and modes of human–robot interaction (voice interaction, tactile interaction via the screen, motion analysis, remote control) are the result of three years of interdisciplinary research using mixed methods: Human–Computer Interface, Software Engineering, Human Factors, Assistive and Rehabilitation Technologies, Human-Centered Design and Participatory Design.

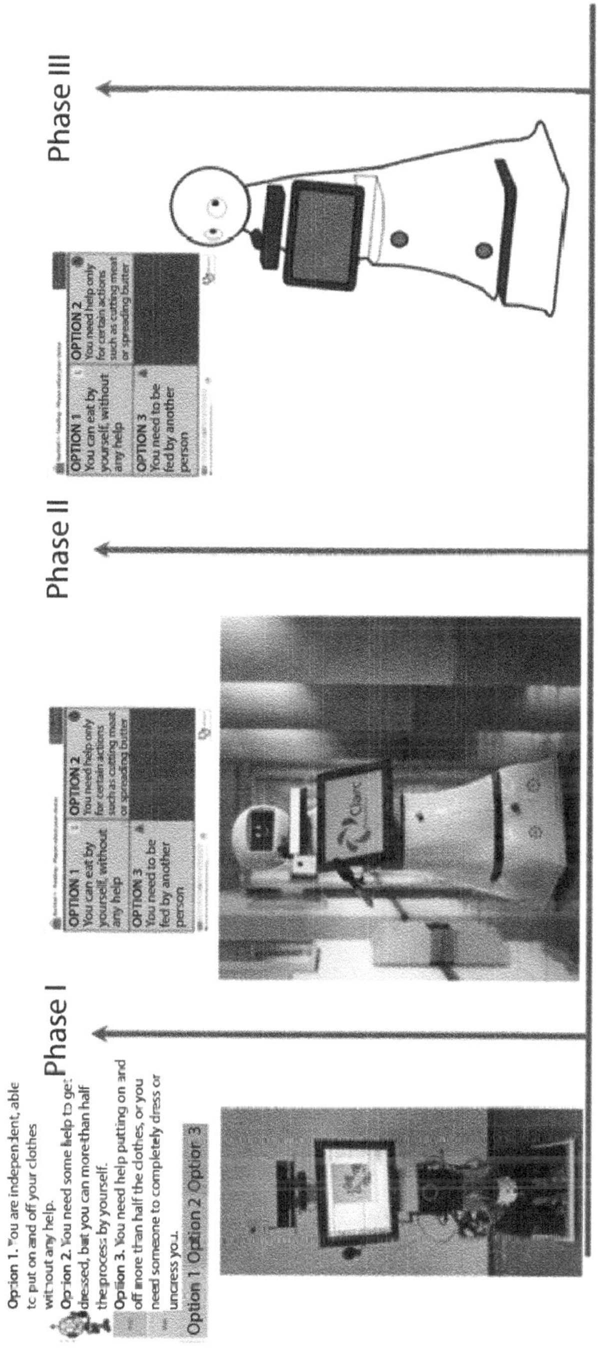

Figure 9.2. *Different iterative phaszes of development*

Consequently, following an iterative methodology, the user (the patient, family caregiver or healthcare professional) was involved throughout the entire design and evaluation processes. The latter participated, in chronological order, in the preliminary user tests examining the acceptability and usability of the robot geriatric assistant (Lan Hing Ting *et al.* 2017), the analysis of comprehensive geriatric assessment practices at the hospital and in particular data collection (Lan Hing Ting *et al.* 2018), the intermediate tests (Iglesias *et al.* forthcoming a.), including the design of specific elements such as improving motion detection (Bandera *et al.* 2017a, 2019), and the co-design of the physical aspect of the robot, up to the pilot assessment in real use situations (presented here in this chapter).

9.2.3. *Hypotheses and research objectives*

On the basis of the knowledge garnered since the start of the project, the research hypothesis, which was recently examined within the framework of this pilot trial, is that a robotic solution would allow for the following efficiency gains in geriatric follow-up (Bandera *et al.* 2016): automated data collection, better saving and sharing of secure data, and better management of caregivers' time on high value-added activities, such as the development of a personalized care plan. This gain in efficiency would allow for an increase in the performance of comprehensive geriatric tests – currently insufficient – of elderly patients for which the demand for treatment is accelerating.

These assumptions, in terms of organizational goals, have been combined with the more practical aspects of the human–robot interaction assessment. In fact, in order to be able to conduct these tests autonomously, the Clara robot must present itself as an assistant who is at once both accessible and useful. Senior citizens undergoing a geriatric assessment are generally unfamiliar with robotic technologies. In addition, age implies decreases in visual, auditory and/or cognitive abilities. It is therefore critical, in terms of social acceptability, that the Clara robot is easy for elderly patients to use, and it must be able to offer more natural, intuitive as well as accessible modes of interaction.

9.3. Methodological approach: living lab approach

With the aim of *empowering* the elderly, the approach adopted throughout this project is the *Living Lab* approach, which combines, among other approaches: iterative design, human-centered design and participatory design. Users – both elderly patients and various experts – were involved throughout the design and iterative evaluation phase, as explained below. The human-centered design would be the human–machine interaction, centered on the exploration of new social practices in our information society (Castells 1998) in and through technologies which give primacy to human actors, to their values and to their activities. It takes human capacities (of the elderly) as a starting point, with an emphasis on how to support the capacities of the elderly through the latest technological developments in assistive technology (Bannon 2011). Participatory design (Kensing and Blomberg 1998) is a cooperative design process, which aims to enable different stakeholders with different perspectives and skills to cooperate. It includes the involvement and active participation of users in the design of the systems they will use (Bratteteig and Wagner 2016). Besides the pragmatic dimension (achieving an acceptable design), the socio-political dimension is also important: the "voice" of future users, who are placed at the center of design concerns, is heard and taken into account, and they have real decision-making power in the design and evaluation of this technology. The notion of empowerment is therefore both an object of reflection and also an objective to be achieved, which guided the development of the AUSUS analytical framework (described below in section 9.3.2).

9.3.1. *Empowerment in and through interaction*

Indeed, the issue of *empowerment*, linked to the interaction of elderly users with the Clara robot assistant, was taken into account in the design phase regarding two considerations. The first aspect concerns the interaction design. As described above, the Clara robot offers four modes of interaction (voice, touch, gesture, physical buttons), and is thus able to adapt to the needs and preferences of each user. Indeed, the remote control was developed during phase 2 (see Figure 9.2) on the basis of the observation (results of successive user tests in France and Spain) that many users encountered significant difficulties in using the voice and touch controls. In addition, the verbal communication for the Clara robot's synthetic voice program contained instructions to mimic a human attitude of benevolence towards its interlocutor: as least authoritative as possible, with pauses allowing for the understanding time as needed by the user. In this way, the hypothesis examined is that the robot assistant Clara would succeed in putting users unfamiliar with robotic technologies at ease, and help to reassure them.

Besides multimodality, the second aspect linked to the empowerment of user interactions with the Clara robot is the accessibility criterion. As discussed previously, age implies decreases in visual, auditory and/or cognitive abilities. The modes of interaction must therefore be natural, intuitive (aspect 1) as well as accessible (aspect 2).

9.3.2. *Contribution: new analytical framework*

As a follow-up to the multimodal interaction design, an analytical framework was specifically developed as part of this research project (Iglesias *et al.* forthcoming b). In order to address the specific characteristics of geriatric patients, the accessibility criterion has been shown to be complementary to the other usual assessment factors. Accessibility, linked to the concepts of "Universal Design" or "Design for All" (Iwarsson and Stahl 2003) in a human–computer interface, has as its main objective the aim of producing systems usable by all, without discrimination, whatever their physical or cognitive capacities (Abascal and Nicolle 2005).

The commonly accepted USUS framework (Weiss *et al.* 2009) allows for the evaluation of humanoid robots used in collaborative tasks. The acronym stands for the following factors – Usability, Social acceptance, User experience, Societal impact. Although representing a useful basis, the USUS framework proved insufficient for this study, due to the profile of the users and the context of use (one-shot test). We have therefore broadened the existing analytical framework of USUS to include the additional criterion of accessibility. Our contribution is thus the AUSUS analytical framework, a mixed methodological framework combining qualitative and quantitative approaches. In this pilot assessment, AUSUS made it possible to evaluate the performance of the robot in carrying out the two tests – *Barthel* and *Get Up & Go* – while examining the efficiency of the human–robot interaction (see the section on results, section 9.4.2, detailed below).

9.3.3. *Mixed methodological approach*

This experiment brings together the characteristics and objectives of both *field trials* (Brown *et al.* 2011; Kjeldskov and Skov 2014), as practiced in the field of human–machine interaction, and *pilot studies* in health research (Van Teijlingen and Hundley 2001; Thabane *et al.* 2010). Hence, it was possible to test this experimental system in an uncontrolled real situation, in a rehabilitation and functional rehabilitation hospital, in a complementary manner to the laboratory usability tests carried out in the previous steps. Thus, the duration of the study – three months – mitigated against the novelty effect (de Graaf *et al.* 2015). Furthermore, this pilot study made it possible to assess the feasibility of another longitudinal study, part of the continuity for this research which began in November 2019 in Andalusia (Iglesias *et al.* 2020).

Aiming for a complementarity of both approaches, the authors adopted a mixed methodological approach (O'Cathain *et al.* 2007) for the research protocol. Defined as integrating the collection and analysis of quantitative and qualitative data in a single study or program (Creswell *et al.* 2004), the complementarity this approach brings to the study is recommended (Pope and Mays 1995). The objective of using this mixed methodological framework is twofold: on the one hand, triangulation, which ensures the validity of quantitative analyses (Östlund *et al.* 2010), and, on the other hand, the complementarity of quantitative and qualitative methodologies, the latter allowing for a more detailed and contextualized understanding of the quantitative results (Pope and Mays 1995). The goal is to produce results that combine credibility with meaning (Guével *et al.* 2016).

Mixed methodology research has been of interest to health researchers for many years. Various combinations of methods have been used in health research in the context of evaluating services, exploring health issues and developing research instruments (O'Cathain *et al.* 2007). They are entering health research practice at the same time as more and more professionals and researchers are convinced of the usefulness of qualitative methods (Guével *et al.* 2016), including those in France.

Accordingly, the AUSUS analytical framework, specifically developed within the framework of this research, is a mix of quantitative (durations, measurement of criteria according to a Lickert scale) and qualitative, combining an interest in what is both *said* (interview) and *done* (ethnographic observation, analysis of the activity through video recordings) throughout the course of the test.

9.4. Pilot assessment

The results presented in this chapter relate to the *Barthel* test with a cohort of 25 patients. As defined by our project consortium partners, ECHORD++ CLARC, based at the *Hospital Universitario Virgen del Rocío* in Seville, the inclusion criteria are: to be at least 65 years of age and to have an MMSE test score greater than or equal to 23. The exclusion criteria are: hearing impairment and visual impairment.

The Barthel test is a 10-question questionnaire on functional abilities. The patient-user can respond in three ways: voice interaction, touch interaction via the screen, or by pressing the buttons on the remote control.

9.4.1. *Procedure and test protocol*

The test is organized as follows. Firstly, the study is presented by the investigator: the patient signs informed consent after being fully informed. Then, a short pre-test questionnaire gauges the level of technology use of the patient-testers, their impression of the robots, as well as any experience with the geriatric test in question. The test itself is videotaped (three complementary viewing angles), for detailed activity analysis, and observed in real time by the investigator, who remains in the room with the patient and the robot (without intervening).

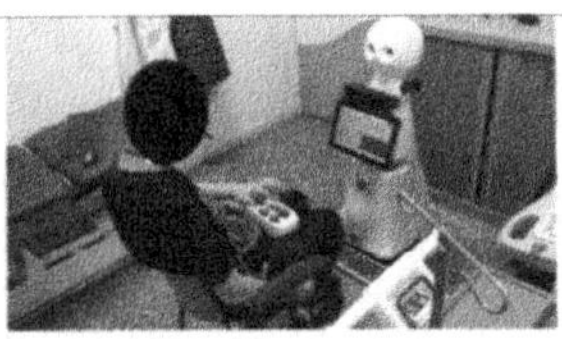	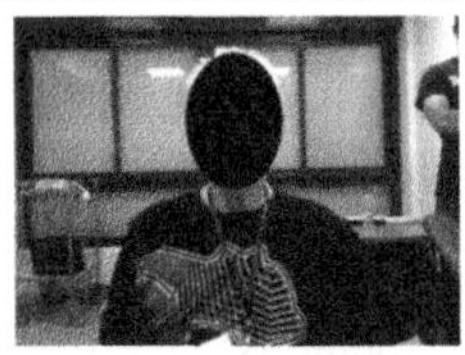	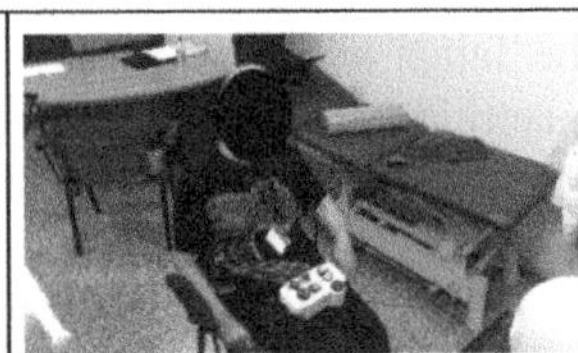
View allowing for the observation of the user's hands, as well as their feet, and possible gestures in relation to the screen of the robot (visible only by this camera).	Located in the robot's eye, this view allows for a clear view of the user's facial expressions.	View to see the tester's facial expressions, as well as the use of the remote control and the gestures they can perform with it.

Figure 9.3. *Different viewing angles to analyze activity*

After the test with the robot, the AUSUS questionnaire guides a semi-structured interview, during which the investigator can deepen certain aspects of interaction in a way that is relevant to the *in situ* observation they have just made.

9.4.2. *Results*

Among the main insights is the preferred mode of interaction, which is the use of the remote control. This preference confirms the intermediate hypothesis that emerged from the user tests in phase 2 of the project, namely the need for an interaction mode other than voice and touch, which would be easier and more accessible for older users.

With the exception of three patients whose durations are below or far below the average (9 min 10 sec, 15 min 35 sec and 14 min 21 sec), the average duration of the tests is 10 minutes (12 tests) or 11 minutes (10 tests).

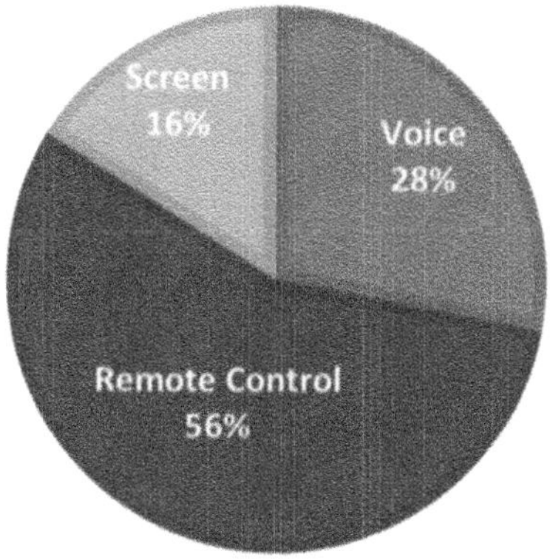

Figure 9.4. *Users' preferred interaction modes*

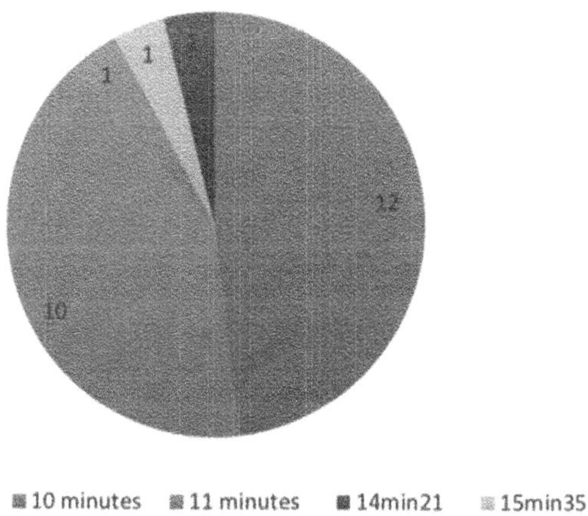

Figure 9.5. *Average test time: 10–11 minutes. The numbers within the circle denote the number of people who took that amount of time*

The system has proven to be robust, with acceptable performance in the face of contingencies: 24 out of 25 patients completed the test (1 in 25 failure rate).

As explained above, the AUSUS analysis framework served as the basis for the evaluation of performance indicators. After the robot interaction session, during a semi-structured interview based on a questionnaire, patients were asked to survey the interaction aspects on a 5-point Lickert scale ranging from 1 (strongly disagree) to 5 (strongly agree).

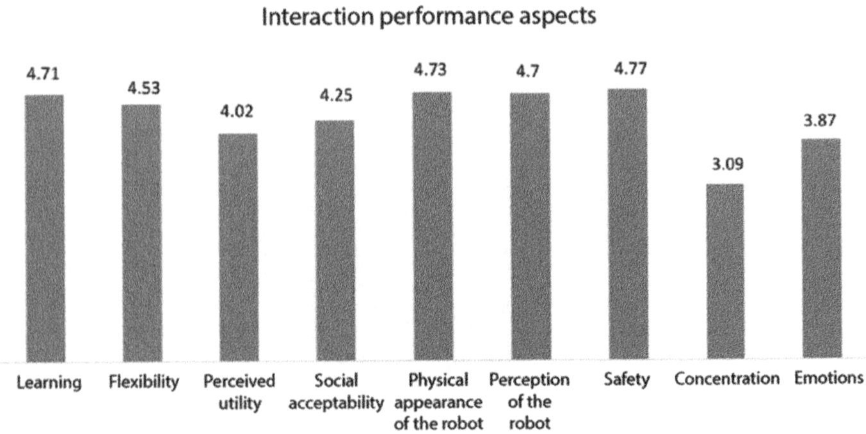

Figure 9.6. *Assessment scores for interaction aspects (out of 5)*

The various aspects of interaction evaluated receive encouraging scores: an average above 4 out of a total of 5 (Learning, Flexibility, Perceived utility, Social acceptability, Physical appearance of the robot, Perception of the robot, Safety), and an average above 3 out of 5 for more complex aspects of human–robot interaction (Concentration, Emotions).

Finally, all the patients said they were satisfied that they took part in this study.

9.5. Conclusion

The understanding generated by this assessment of operations in real-world situations served, in a pragmatic way, to inform the design of the robot within the framework of an iterative improvement, concerning: the interface, the voice interaction, the intelligibility of instructions, and motion detection. Due to the duration of the experiment, the novelty effect (de Graaf *et al.* 2015) could be avoided. Even if the actual use during the test was unique (one-shot), the robot's regular presence at the rehabilitation center allowed for the necessary familiarization. In addition, a form of social acceptability seems to appear in the ethnographic survey data through the positive attitude of some of the patients and staff at this hospital center to the presence of the interactive robot.

The insights gained were also used to evaluate and improve the AUSUS analytical framework, which was implemented by this pilot assessment, in view of its broader application. In particular, this experiment confirms the advantages of a mixed methodological approach, combining a quantitative approach that allows for an objectification of the results, with a qualitative approach that makes it possible to make better sense of them. The benefits of this approach are further confirmed by research in health, the human–computer interface, and even more so for something as complex and new as human–robot interaction.

From a methodological and reflective perspective, the knowledge generated by this pilot experiment is also used to nourish reflection concerning the future deployment of such a fully functional technological tool in a longitudinal clinical study (ROSI and ITERA projects which constitute the work following on from ECHORD ++ CLARC, see Iglesias *et al.* 2020). Indeed, for Van Teijlingen and Hundley (2001), pilot studies are a crucial component of good study design. As such, they encourage researchers to report on it, especially on improvements made to the study design and research process. This is precisely the objective of the authors' contribution in this chapter.

9.6. Acknowledgments

This work was partially funded by the *European Clearing House for Open Robotics Development Plus Plus* project (ECHORD++ CLARC (FP7-ICT-601116)). The authors warmly thank their colleagues from the CLARC consortium, Guillaume Beghin, M1 trainee at the Living Lab ActivAgeing, the team from the *Centre Hospitalier de Troyes*, Professor Jean-Luc Novella from the *CHU de Reims*, their colleagues – Philippe Voisin, Guillaume Dessinger and Matthieu Detroy – and especially the patients of the *CRRF COS Pasteur*, for their participation in this research.

9.7. References

Abascal, J. and Nicolle, C. (2005). Moving towards inclusive design guidelines for socially and ethically aware HCI. *Interacting with Computers*, 17(5), 484–505.

Bandera, A., Bandera, J.P., Bustos, P., Calderita, L.V., Duenas, A., Fernandez, F., Fuentetaja, R., Garcia-Olaya, A., Francisco, F., Garcia-Polo, F.J., Gonzalez, J.C., Iglesias, A., Manso, L.J., Marfil, R., Pulido, J.C., Reuther, C., Romero-Garces, A., Suarez, C. (2016). CLARC: A robotic architecture for comprehensive geriatric assessment. *Proceedings of the WAF 2016*, June.

Bandera, J.P., Romero-Garces, A., Duenas, A., Marfil, R., Lan Hing Ting, K., Voilmy, D., Garcia-Polo, F.J. (2017a). Towards autonomous gait analysis in the Get Up and Go test. In *REACTS 2017, 4th Workshop on Recognition and Action for Scene Understanding*, Azzopardi, J.D.G. and Marfil, R. (eds). Creative Commons, Mountain View, CA.

Bandera, A., Bandera, J.P., Barile, T., Bustos, P., Calderita, L.V., Duenas, A., Fernandez, F., Fuentetaja, R., Garcia-Olaya, A., Garcia, J., Gonzalez, J.C., Iglesias, A., Lan Hing Ting, K., Manso, L.J., Marfil, R., Pulido, J.C., Reuther, C., Romero-Garces, A., Suarez, C., Voilmy, D. (2017b). CLARC: A cognitive robot for helping geriatric doctors in real scenarios, *ROBOT'2017 – 3rd Iberian Robotics Conference*, Seville, 22–24 November.

Bandera, J.P., Marfil, R., Romero-Garces, A., Voilmy, D. (2019). A new paradigm for autonomous human motion description and evaluation: Application to the Get Up & Go test use case. *Pattern Recognition Letters*, 118, 51–60.

Bannon, L. (2011) Reimagining HCI: Toward a more human-centered perspective. *Interactions*, 18(4), 50–57.

Bratteteig, T. and Wagner, I. (2016). Unpacking the notion of participation in participatory design. *Computer Supported Cooperative Work*, 25(6), 425–475.

Broekens, J., Heerink, M., Rosendal, H. (2009). Assistive social robots in elderly care: A review. *Gerontechnology*, 8(2), 94–103.

Brown, B., Reeves, S., Sherwood, S. (2011). Into the wild: Challenges and opportunities for field trial methods. *Proceedings of the SIGCHI Conference on Human Factors in Computing Systems (CHI '11)*. ACM, New York.

Castells, M. (1998). *L'ère de l'information I. La société en réseaux*, translated by Philippe Delamare. Fayard, Paris.

Creswell, J.W., Fetters, M.D., Ivankova, N.V. (2004). Designing a mixed methods study in primary care. *Annals of Family Medicine*, 2, 7–12.

Feil-Seifer, D. and Matarić, M. (2005). Defining socially assistive robotics. *Proceedings of the International Conference on Rehabilitation Robotics (ICORR)*, Chicago, IL.

de Graaf, M.M.A., Ben Allouch, S., Klamer, T. (2015). Sharing a life with Harvey: Exploring the acceptance of and relationship-building with a social robot. *Computers in Human Behavior*, 43, 1–14.

Guével, M.R., Pommier, J., Absil, G. (2016). Articuler des méthodes qualitatives et quantitatives – illustrations de la conceptualisation par les méthodes mixtes. In *Les recherches qualitatives en santé*, Kivits, J., Ballard, F., Fournier, C., Winance, M. (eds). Armand Colin, Paris.

Iglesias, A., Viciana-Abad, R., Perez-Lorenzo, J.M., Lan Hing Ting, K., Tudela, A., Marfil, R., Duenas, A., Bandera, J.P. (2020). Towards long-term acceptance of socially assistive robots in retirement houses: Use case definition. *Proceedings of the 2020 IEEE International Conference on Autonomous Robot Systems and Competitions (ICARSC)*, Ponta Delgada, 15–17 April.

Iglesias, A., Garcia, A., Garcia-Olaya, A., Fuentetaja, R., Fernandez, F., Romero-Garces, A., Marfil, R., Bandera, A., Lan Hing Ting, K., Voilmy, D., Duenas A., Suarez, C. (forthcoming a). Influence of the patient-robot interaction on the accuracy of robotized geriatric assessments. *International Journal of Social Robotics*.

Iglesias, A., Garcia, A., Garcia-Olaya, A., Fuentetaja, R., Fernandez, F., Romero-Garces, A., Marfil, R., Bandera, A., Lan Hing Ting, K., Voilmy, D., Duenas, A., Suarez, C. (forthcoming b). Extending the evaluation of social robots with accessibility indicators. The AUSUS evaluation framework. *IEEE Transactions on Human-Machine Systems*.

Iwarsson, S. and Stahl, A. (2003). Accessibility, usability and universal design positioning and definition of concepts describing person-environment relationships. *Disability and Rehabilitation*, 25(2), 57–66.

Kensing, F. and Blomberg, J. (1998). Participatory design: Issues and concerns. *Computer Supported Cooperative Work (CSCW)*, 7, 167–185.

Kjeldskov, J. and Skov, M.B. (2014). Was it worth the hassle? Ten years of mobile HCI research discussions on lab and field evaluations. *MobileHCI '14: Proceedings of the 16th International Conference on Human-Computer Interaction with Mobile Devices and Service*. Association for Computing Machinery, New York.

Lan Hing Ting, K., Voilmy, D., Iglesias, A., Pulido, J.C., Garcia, J., Romero-Garces, A., Bandera, J.P., Marfil, R., Duenas, A. (2017). Integrating the users in the design of a robot for making comprehensive geriatric assessments (CGA) to elderly people in care centers. *IEEE RO-MAN2017, 26th IEEE International Symposium on Robot and Human Interactive Communication*, Lisbon, 28 August–1 September.

Lan Hing Ting, K., Voilmy, D., Iglesias, A., Marfil, R. (2018). Data collection in CGA evaluation: Analyzing clinicians' practices to inform design. *Workshop Data Work in Healthcare 2018, CSCW 2018 – The 21st ACM Conference on Computer-supported Cooperative Work and Social Computing*, New York City's Hudson River, 3–7 November.

Matthews, D.A. (1984). Dr. Marjory Warren and the origin of the British geriatrics. *Journal of the American Geriatrics Society*, 34, 253–258.

Nevejans, N. (2017). *Traité de droit et d'éthique de la robotique civile*. LEH Édition, Bordeaux.

Nord, M., Lyth, J., Alwin, J., Marcusson, J. (2021). Costs and effects of comprehensive geriatric assessment in primary care for older adults with high risk for hospitalisation. *BMC Geriatrics*, 21(1), 263, April 21.

O'Cathain, A., Murphy, E., Nicholl, J. (2007). Why, and how, mixed methods research is undertaken in health services research: A mixed methods study. *BMC Health Services Research*, 7, 85.

O'Cathain A., Nicholl, J., Murphy, E. (2009). Structural issues affecting mixed methods studies in health research: A qualitative study. *BMC Medical Research Methodology*, 9, 82.

Östlund, U., Kidd, L., Wengstrom, Y., Rowa-Dewar, N. (2010). Combining qualitative and quantitative research within mixed method research designs: A methodological review. *Int. J. Nurs. Stud.*, 48, 369–383, doi:10.1016/j.ijnurstu.2010.10.005.

Pope, C. and Mays, N. (1995). Qualitative research: Reaching the parts other methods cannot reach: An introduction to qualitative methods in health and health services research. *BMJ*, 311, 42–45.

Stuck, A.E., Siu, A.L., Wieland, G.D., Adams, J., Rubenstein, L.Z. (1993). Comprehensive geriatric assessment: A meta-analysis of controlled trials. *Lancet*, 342, 1032.

Thabane, L., Ma, J., Chu, R., Cheng, J., Ismaila, A., Rios, L.P., Robson, R., Thabane, M., Giangregorio, L., Goldsmith, C.H. (2010). A tutorial on pilot studies: The what, why and how. *BMC Med. Res. Methodol.*, 10, 1.

Turner, G. and Clegg, A. (2014). Best practice guidelines for the management of frailty: A British Geriatrics Society. *Age UK and Royal College of General Practitioners Report, Age Ageing*, 43(6), 744–777.

Van Teijlingen, E.R. and Hundley, V. (2001). The importance of pilot studies. *Social Research Update*, 35 [Online]. Available at: http://sru.soc.surrey.ac.uk/SRU35.html.

Voilmy, D., Suárez, C., Romero-Garcés, A., Reuther, C., Pulido, J.C., Marfil, R., Manso, L.J., Lan Hing Ting, K., Iglesias, A., González, J.C., García, J., García-Olaya, A., Fuentetaja, R., Fernández, F., Dueñas, A., Calderita, L.V., Bustos, P., Barile, T., Bandera, J.P., Bandera, A. (2017). CLARC: A cognitive robot for helping geriatric doctors in real scenarios. In *ROBOT 2017: Third Iberian Robotics Conference : Advances in Intelligent Systems and Computing*, Ollero, A., Sanfeliu, A., Montano, L., Lau, N., Cardeira, C. (eds). Springer, Cham.

Weiss, A., Bernhaupt, R., Lankes, M., Tscheligi, M. (2009). The USUS evaluation framework for human-robot interaction. *AISB2009: Proceedings of the Symposium on New Frontiers in Human-Robot Interaction*, 158–165.

10

Perspectives on the Patient Experience (PX) of People with Disabilities in the Digital Age: From UX to PX

10.1. Introduction

User-centered approaches, in the sense of Norman (1986, pp. 31–61) or of the ISO 9241-210: 2019 standard, now need to be systematically used for any design or improvement of healthcare systems. It is important that the patient is considered as a real actor with regard to their own healthcare journey. In addition, it is also important to provide easy access to the hospital's digital services and optimizing the flow of information between the different hubs or health sectors, and therefore between different actors within the organization. These accesses are relevant in different contexts: before, during and after the care of the patient, in order to allow patients to have, in particular, a good digital experience or an adapted way of living with technology. This is generally called User eXperience (UX), which has been the subject of much research and many proposals (Alben 1996; Hassenzahl and Tractinsky 2006). This digital experience concerns doctors, nursing and hospital staff, patients, caregivers, partners and health service institutions. This is referred to as the Patient eXperience or PX (AHRQ 2017).

A problem arises concerning patients with disabilities (AHRQ 2019), whose needs are specific, and can widely vary according to their kind of disability. These patients can live very restrictive and different digital experiences. Different categories of questions arise: what sorts of access devices and what services could be put in place to improve the experience of this category of patients? For example,

---

Chapter written by Djilali IDOUGHI, Karim TOULOUM, Yohan GUERRIER and Christophe KOLSKI.

making an appointment and going to the hospital can cause different types of problems depending on the nature of the disability. In addition, when a patient arrives at the hospital, when a patient arrives, they usually have to take a ticket at a terminal. This action sounds simple for an able-bodied person, but may be difficult for a person with a motor impairment.

In this regard, within the field of disability, the numerous disabilities are organized into several categories: physical, mental and psychological (Winance 2008). Each category is usually made up of dozens of different disabilities, each with its own characteristics. Each person with a disability therefore has specific needs in relation to the systems to be used. For example, a blind person will not have the same needs as an upper or lower limb amputee. It is therefore important to take UX in general into account, and Patient eXperience (PX) in particular for our case, in the design of an interactive system or a health process that includes digital services. However, sometimes, collecting information on user needs encounters implementation difficulties for the design of systems dedicated to people with disabilities with different types of disabilities: communication, motor, cognitive, etc. (Antona *et al.* 2009, pp. 15-1–15-14).

In this chapter, we deal with the dimension of the digitization of the healthcare journey, aiming to experience it as it is by a patient with a disability. This refers, in part, to the web accessibility initiative (WAI n.d), as web services can help improve health journeys. This presents a set of challenges, which relate to the technical and methodological preparations to be considered when developing digital services that are focused on patients with disabilities and which must be dealt with as early as possible (Altinier 2012). It is with this in mind that we propose a first approach to developing this patient experience which will integrate the various stakeholders (patients, accompanying persons, hospital or medical staff, and health professionals), while identifying new uses linked to the healthcare journey of patients with disabilities.

This approach aims to take into account the web accessibility recommendations and criteria described by the Web Content Accessibility Guidelines (WCAG n.d), User Agent Accessibility Guidelines (UAAG n.d) and Authoring Tool Accessibility Guidelines (ATAG n.d).

10.2. State-of-the-art on Patient eXperience (PX)

UX, for which examples of implementation can be found in numerous documents, including those of Gube (2010), Touloum *et al.* (2012) and (Komminos 2019), deals with the way in which a user interacts with a system and how this experience is felt. In this area, there are many ways to gather information about UX, such as through questionnaires or focus groups (Lallemand and Gronier 2018).

As we can see in Figure 10.1, adapted from Lallemand and Gronier (2018), in general, the design of an application or a good takes place in several stages. Stage 1 is the planning stage (the definition of the objectives of a project and reflection on the tools and resources necessary). Stage 2 is devoted to exploration (collecting information on user needs). Stage 3 is the ideation phase (summary of the exploration phase and production of ideas for the design). The purpose of stage 4 is generation (the formalization of design solution(s)). Lastly, stage 5 is devoted to the iterative evaluation of the solutions generated. We can clearly see in Figure 10.1 that this process is iterative: this means that there are usually several back-and-forths between the different phases. Thanks to these back-and-forths, the designer places the future user at the center of development in order to better meet the requirements.

More specifically, in the area of disability and user-centered design, the aim is to highlight an important theme to determine the ecosystem of the person with a disability. Depending on the case and the type of disability, the ecosystem may be composed of the disabled person using the system, the accompanying person, who may be either a family member or a professional, different people with whom they will be interacting or the likely assistance tools; this ecosystem can vary enormously depending on the context (Guffroy *et al.* 2017, 2018, pp. 462–465; Sauzin 2017). Ecosystem actors can often help define the user's needs for the design of their future system(s). To better understand this, we cite the communication aid called ComMob (Guerrier 2015) as an example. This software tool was developed by the third author of this chapter: Yohan Guerrier. It allows sentences to be formulated from pictograms which are organized by category and theme. In this case, the ecosystem was made up of the user, their caregiver and ComMob, as well as various counterparts, known or unknown *a priori*, which may vary depending on the context (e.g. if the user has mobility). During the development of this application, the needs of the user were expressed both by the designer, who is himself disabled, and by various caregivers; field evaluations were also carried out in the presence of interlocutors unknown *a priori* (Guerrier *et al.* 2014, pp. 419–426).

After defining the UX theme, it is time to apply it to the medical field. PX (AHRQ 2017) includes all of the interactions that patients can have with a healthcare system and may include their doctors, nurses, healthcare practitioners, etc. As an integral component of the healthcare quality system, PX includes several aspects of healthcare delivery that patients expect when seeking and receiving care, such as scheduling appointments, accessing information and better communication with their interlocutors, wherever they are located, both inside and outside health establishments.

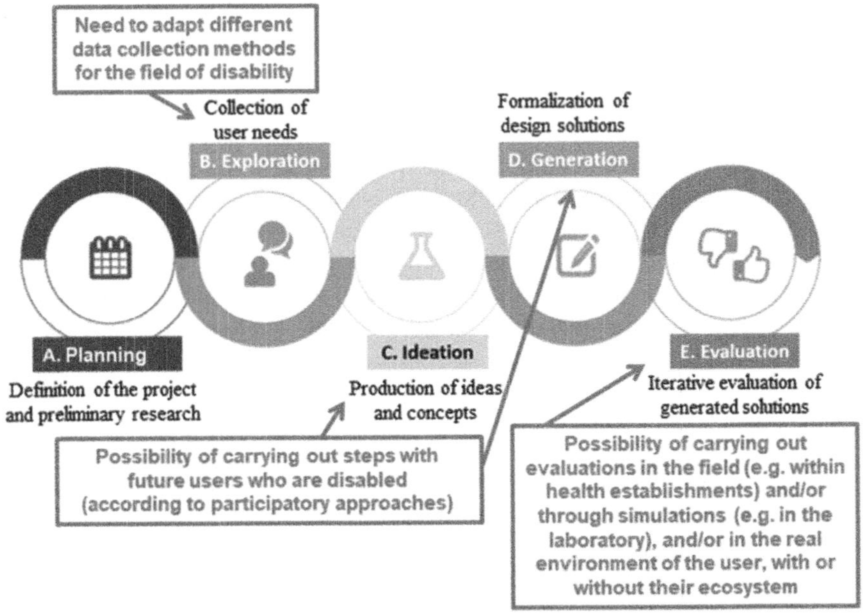

Figure 10.1. *Iterative design cycle of interactive systems (adapted from Lallemand and Gronier 2018, with various additions in green related to the field of disability). For a color version of this figure, see www.iste.co.uk/chaabane/healthcare.zip*

Disabled patients for whom the PX is different and restrictive require an adapted approach to meet their specific needs, in conjunction with appropriate digital services. Thus, when we consider the different aspects of PX, we can assess the extent to which patients receive associated care and services that are appropriate and customizable to individual characteristics, preferences, needs and expectations. In addition, evaluating PX with other components, such as the efficiency and safety of healthcare, is essential in order to convey a holistic view of the quality of care being provided. Therefore, understanding PX is a key step towards patient-centered healthcare. Various methods for collecting information on PX are provided by the specialized literature; see, for example, the Consumer Assessment of Healthcare Providers and Systems (CAHPS) (AHRQ 2017).

In recent years, a growing interest from academia and industry has enriched the concept of PX, placing greater import on it with regard to the constant endeavor to improve the quality of healthcare provided and reduce costs. PX is becoming a key factor in the healthcare revolution. On the other hand, little tangible field work has been undertaken in PX in the digital age. To this end, the objective of the digital transformation of the patient journey through all assistive technologies (Altinier 2012, 2019; W3C 2017) is to ensure the continuity and improvement of care at each stage of the patient journey. This journey has been enhanced thanks to the associated digital tools, by means of multiplatform access, capable of improving the PX, on the one hand, and of modifying the practices of healthcare professionals, on the other, as shown in Figure 10.2.

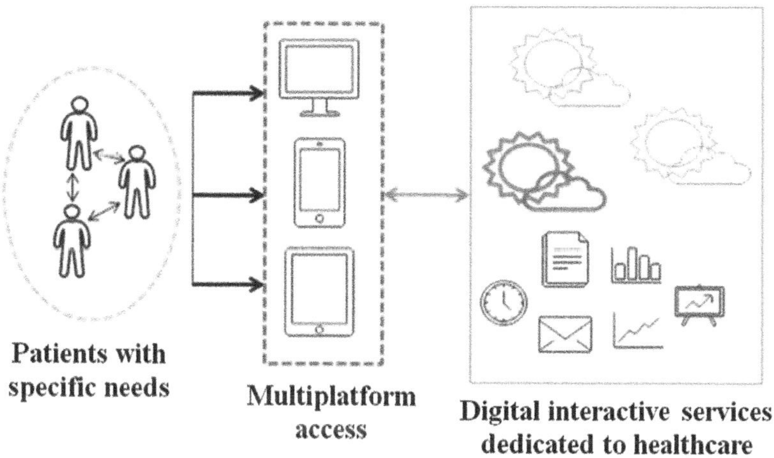

Figure 10.2. *General view of the digital health concept. For a color version of this figure, see www.iste.co.uk/chaabane/healthcare.zip*

10.3. Research methodology and proposal

The aim is to propose a methodological framework (see Figure 10.3) for the development of the PX for people with specific needs during their care journey, while taking into account the recommendations and criteria for web accessibility stated in WCAG2, adapted from W3C (W3C 2017) and AccessiWeb (Altinier 2019). While retaining common concepts with classic user centered design, according to Norman (1986, pp. 31–61, 2013), or the ISO standard[1], in participatory

1 Where the needs, expectations and specific characteristics of the end users are taken into account at each step of the product development process. This approach is based on the idea that the end users are best placed to express their own needs, and thus should participate in the design, evaluation and use of the interactive system, up until the needs and requirements expressed by these users are satisfied.

design (Schuler and Namioka 1993; Kensing 2003) and the "Design for All" approach (Stephanidis and Salvendy 1998; Stephanidis 2001), the idea is to go a little further, we are not focusing on the system but on a complete journey, considering very different situations, from the points of view of a set of actors, and possibly requiring a set of systems. In each situation to be taken into account, the ecosystem of the patient with a disability will be considered, paying close attention (as emphasized above).

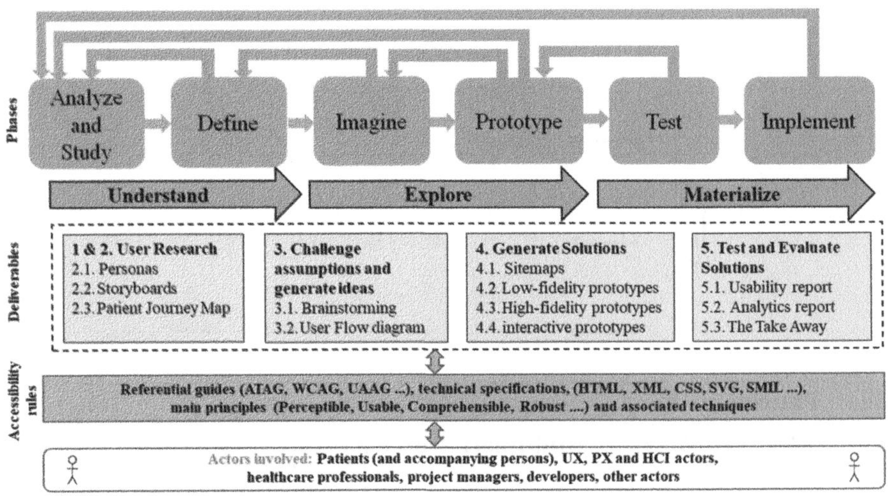

Figure 10.3. *Global view of the development methodological framework (inspired and adapted from Gibbons (2016)). For a color version of this figure, see www.iste.co.uk/chaabane/healthcare.zip*

The conceptual framework is based on the Design Thinking approach, which is an innovation management method, promoting so-called creative or collaborative design, based on a (non-linear) process of co-creativity involving the end user; see, for example, Gibbons (2016), Interaction Design Foundation (n.d), KLAP (2016) and d.school (n.d). Referring to Gibbons (2016), it follows the overall direction to "Understand, Explore, and Materialize" and is broken down into six phases: (1) Analyze and Study, (2) Define, (3) Imagine, (4) Prototype, (5) Test and (6) Implement. The UX deliverables (Komminos 2019) of each phase may vary, depending on the roles of the project team, on the one hand, and on the methods and tools used by each role, on the other (Figure 10.3). The actors who can be involved in the process of developing and delivering the PX for people with specific needs, with a focus on quality, can be greatly varied depending on the healthcare journey concerned, including. in addition to patients (and their possible companions, members of their ecosystem) and actors encountered on the journey (medical secretaries, health personnel, etc.), specialists in UX, PX and human–computer interaction (HCI), members of software development teams and other various players from different fields (marketing, insurance, security, etc.) (see Figure 10.3).

The first two phases, generally grouped under the term "User Research", consist of acquiring a deeper understanding of the problem(s) and needs to be resolved in relation to the profiles of the actors concerned. The deliverables of this phase can be visualized and synthesized through different types of methods taken from the UX field: personas (Cooper 1999; Seffah *et al.* 2009, pp. 333–336; Brangier and Bornet 2011, pp. 38–61; Idoughi *et al.* 2012; Göltz 2014), storyboards (Krause 2018) and the *Patient Journey Map* approach, the latter being directly derived from the *Customer Journey Map* (or *Experience Map*) approach (Shostack 1977; Komminos 2019). Note that other UX methods could be used, as illustrated by Lallemand and Gronier (2018).

10.4. Illustrations relating to the "user research" phase of the methodological framework

In the "user research" phase of the methodological framework, we propose to first use the Persona technique, situated upstream of other patient-centered research methods, in order to understand the specific or underlying needs of people with disabilities. and their modes of using the web and associated digital technologies. This is an essential prerequisite to meeting the accessibility standards, in the broad sense, for all types of patient journey.

Starting from the principle that it is based on a set of personas covering a representative set of categories of disabled persons, Figure 10.4 illustrates a persona characterized by a data set relating to their disability situation, such as cerebral palsy, expressing their motivations, objectives, needs and expectations in relation to the use of digital technology in the context of their healthcare strategy, while highlighting their constraints and obstacles.

Next, by considering disability as a source of innovation, it is possible to proceed through storyboards (Krause 2018) through which the actions of the user and the circumstances in which they are carried out are described or represented (Figure 10.5).

An eXperience Map is a diagram representing the steps in the process undertaken by the user in order to accomplish a task or to achieve a goal (Komminos 2019). This will allow the designer to understand the changes in terms of the context, in addition to the motivations, issues and needs encountered throughout the process, as illustrated in the case study below.

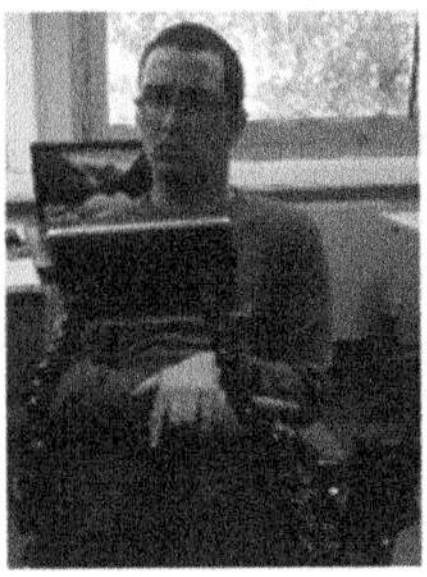

Alain interacting with the tablet installed on his wheelchair

Alain is a researcher in the field of Marine Biology. He works in a laboratory located in Hauts-de-France, a region of France. He is 42 years old, married and the father of 2 children.

Alain uses a communication aid on a daily basis, consisting of pictogram-based software accessed via the tablet on his wheelchair. Alain has cerebral palsy and as such makes involuntary movements, limited in number and low in terms of intensity.

His goal has always been to communicate as easily as possible with those around him, during both personal and professional interactions. According to him, you cannot be integrated into society if you do not have the ability to communicate easily. Thanks to his communication aid, he can organize meetings within the laboratory with his colleagues, even in different languages.

On a personal level, Alain has always had difficulty making medical appointments due to his speech impediments and needs to ask a third party in order to call a doctor. In addition, during the meetings, he must be accompanied so that his remarks can be repeated to the professional. Finally, Alain cannot pay for the consultations himself because of his involuntary movements.

Alain has encountered difficulties throughout his life as a result of his disability. The medical profession often mistakes him for a person with a mental disability. The doctor speaks to the person accompanying him instead of speaking directly to Alain.

In this context, Alain would like specific IT help from the medical field to enable him to communicate directly with the practitioner on his own. In addition, he would like a tool that would allow him to make his own medical appointments, without going through an intermediary.

Figure 10.4. *Persona: Alain. For a color version of this figure, see www.iste.co.uk/chaabane/healthcare.zip*

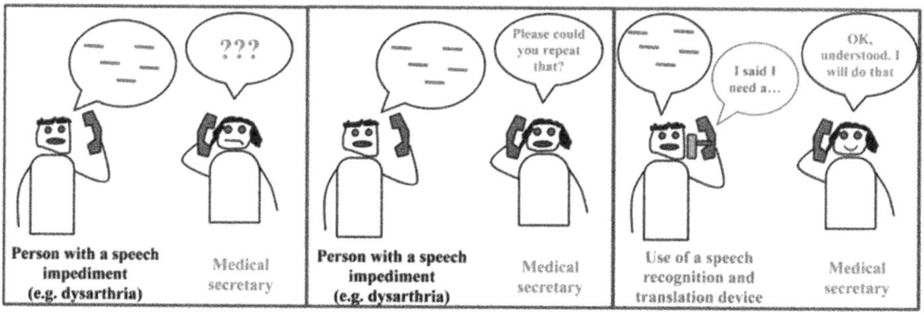

Figure 10.5. *Principle of holistic visualization through storyboards of the actions of disabled persons and the technological/digital environment in which they can take place, with a view to orient towards design choices/decision-making. For a color version of this figure, see www.iste.co.uk/chaabane/healthcare.zip*

10.5. Case study: digital care journey of a patient with a disability

PX journey mapping is a technique for understanding the motivations, needs, hesitations and concerns of patients. It uses visuals and narratives to illustrate the different relationships and interactions that a patient can have with a digital service over a period of time. The narration is expressed from the point of view of the patient, who, for our example, is disabled; this patient describes in detail his experience with the digital service offered. This narration helps the project/development team to concretely and holistically observe the healthcare journey of a patient. The PX journey is organized into stages, each representing a particular goal that the patient with a disability wants to achieve along their healthcare journey. The steps correspond to a goal-oriented and non-process-oriented healthcare journey. Therefore, in order to create the PX Map, we need to consider some relevant questions, such as: (1) How do patients behave in a situation upstream of the implementation of the proposed solution or service? (2) What is the patient problem to be solved, in other words, what are the critical or constraining points that the patient wants to see improved or overcome? (3) How can we improve patient engagement through various communication channels and digital media? Depending on the context and type of disability concerned, the use of a communication support system may be necessary; for further reading on this subject and the different system categories of this type, see Guerrier *et al.* (2018).

The uses linked to the healthcare journey for patients with disabilities may concern patients and caregivers as well as hospital or medical staff; remember that we can also speak of the ecosystem of the disabled person, as described by Guffroy *et al.* (2017), mentioned above. For example, the PX services can be as follows: (1) Messaging services (medical team messages, upstream or downstream healthcare messages, other messages, etc.), (2) Alert services (receiving medication reminders, making an appointment, etc.), (3) Planning and diary services (management of appointments, planning, etc.), (4) Instruction and training services (help with training or education) and (5) Emergency healthcare notifications, etc. In fact, all the services listed above correspond to the different points of contact that the patient may encounter when interacting with their real and digital environments. A very simplified example of an eXperience map, illustrating the patient journey desire to make their own monthly appointment for a medical check-up, is provided by the graphic shown in Figure 10.6; see Lallemand and Gronier (2018) for more detailed illustrations.

The patient achieves a particular goal at the end of each step of the healthcare journey corresponding to the contact points of the following services: (1) contacting consultation services, (2) consideration of the list of doctors after diagnosis, (3) discussion with medical professionals and (4) making an appointment with a suitable doctor. Once the goals and points of contact have been identified and understood, and each stage of the CXP has been covered with the project team, we must successfully identify the potential points of friction and possible difficulties that have or may be encountered and which must be resolved, with a view to improving PX.

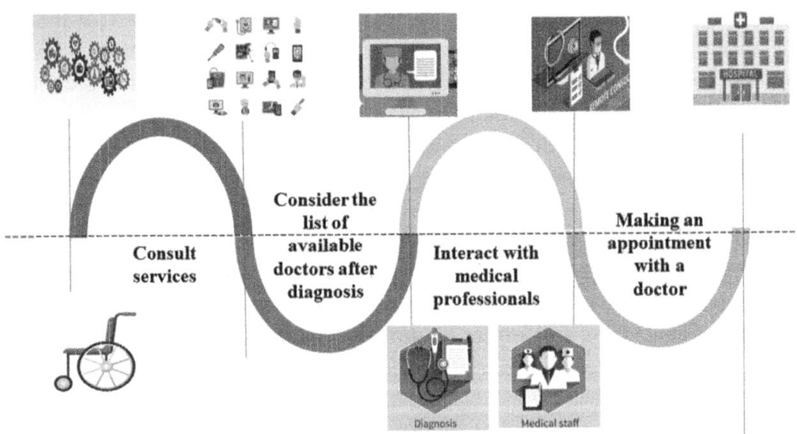

Figure 10.6. *Example of an eXperience map for an "appointment book" patient journey (inspired by Lee* et al. *2015, pp. 66–74; Touloum* et al. *2018; Touloum 2019). For a color version of this figure, see www.iste.co.uk/chaabane/healthcare.zip*

10.6. Conclusion

We have described and positioned the importance of the PX in a patient-centered development approach aiming for an advanced medical management of a patient. We have focused on patients with disabilities for whom the PX may be different and constraining, requiring an adapted approach in order to link their specific needs with the appropriate digital services. Our approach is primarily based on the Design Thinking approach, which is appropriate for the type of problem we are dealing with in this research. It is an innovative methodology that transforms ideas and projects into real activities and tangible prototypes. Certain challenges, in particular those facing UX designers, graphic designers, project managers or even software engineers, may arise, on the one hand, while on the other, opportunities for patients with specific needs, as well as their associated healthcare professionals and medical staff, may also be encountered and taken advantage of.

Each phase of the process is iterative and cyclical as opposed to being a strictly linear process. We can also go back to the first two phases, "Analyze and Study" and "Define", after the development and testing of the initial prototype. Several illustrations associated with the methodological approach have been provided, thus giving a representative overview of the richness and potential of the approach.

There are many research perspectives. Indeed, given the issues formulated in the form of scenarios related to health and, more particularly, to patient journeys, in its interaction with various people involved in the rapid development of the first digital PX services, it is now a question of highlighting the application of this approach in the form of workshops. These would have both design and evaluation goals focusing on the improvement of patient pathways, wherein the participants would try to make the innovative ideas expressed concrete and test them with disabled persons and their possible companions (actors within their ecosystem), in the context of real or simulated situations.

10.7. References

AHRQ (2017). What is patient experience? *Agency for Healthcare Research and Quality*, Rockville [Online]. Available at: https://www.ahrq.gov/cahps/about-cahps/patient-experience/index.html.

AHRQ (2019). About CAHPS. *Agency for Healthcare Research and Quality*, Rockville [Online]. Available at: https://www.ahrq.gov/cahps/about-cahps/index.html [Accessed April 2019].

Alben, L. (1996). Quality of experience: Defining the criteria for effective interaction design. *Interactions*, 3(3), 11–15.

Altinier, A. (2012). *Accessibilité Web : normes et bonnes pratiques pour des sites plus accessibles*. Editions Eyrolles, Paris.

Altinier, A. (2019). Les normes pour l'accessibilité numérique. *Enjeux numériques*, 5, March Annales des Mines, Paris.

Antona, M., Ntoa, S., Adami, I., Stephanidis, C. (2009). User requirements elicitation for universal access. In *The Universal Access Handbook*, Stephanidis, C. (ed.). CRC Press, Boca Raton.

ATAG (n.d). Authoring Tool Accessibility Guidelines (ATAG) overview [Online]. Available at: https://www.w3.org/WAI/standards-guidelines/atag/.

Augusto, J., Kramer, D., Alegre, U., Covaci, A., Santokhee, A. (2018). The user-centred intelligent environments development process as a guide to co-create smart technology for people with special needs. *Universal Access in Information Society*, 17, 115–130.

Brangier, E. and Bornet, C. (2011). Persona: A method to produce representations focused on consumers' needs. In *Human Factors and Ergonomics in Consumer Product Design*, Karwowski, W., Soares, M., Stanton, N. (eds). Taylor and Francis, Boca Raton.

Cooper, A. (1999). *The Inmates are Running the Asylum*. SAMS Publishing, Indianapolis.

d.school (n.d) d.school [Online]. Available at: https://dschool.stanford.edu/.

Gibbons, S. (2016). Design thinking. *Nielsen Norman Group* [Online]. Available at: https://www.nngroup.com/articles/design-thinking/.

Göltz, S. (2014). A closer look at personas: What they are and how they work 1. *Smashing Magazine* [Online]. Available at: https://www.smashingmagazine.com/2014/08/a-closer-look-at-personas-part-1/.

Gube, J. (2010). What is user experience design? Overview, tools and resources. *Smashing Magazine* [Online]. Available at: https://www.smashingmagazine.com/2010/10/what-is-user-experience-design-overview-tools-and-resources/.

Guerrier, Y. (2015). Proposition d'une aide logicielle pour la saisie d'information en situation dégradée – application à des utilisateurs IMC athétosiques dans des contextes liés au transport et aux activités journalières. PhD Thesis, Université de Valenciennes et du Hainaut-Cambrésis, Valenciennes.

Guerrier, Y., Naveteur, J., Kolski, C., Poirier, F. (2014). Communication system for persons with cerebral palsy – *In situ* observation of social interaction following assisted information request. In *Proceedings of ICCHP 2014: Computers Helping People with Special Needs – 14th International Conference, Part I,* Miesenberger, K., Fels, D., Archambault, D., Peňáz, P., Zagler, W. (eds). LNCS, Springer, Cham.

Guerrier, Y., Kolski, C., Poirier, F. (2018). État de l'art sur les systèmes d'aide à la communication envisageables pour des utilisateurs de profil IMC athétosique. *Journal d'interaction personne-système*, 6(1), 1–45.

Guffroy, M., Vigouroux, N., Kolski, C., Vella, F., Teutsch, P. (2017). From human-centered design to disabled user and ecosystem centered design in case of assistive interactive systems. *International Journal of Sociotechnology and Knowledge Development*, 9(4), 28–42.

Guffroy, M., Guerrier, Y., Kolski, C., Vigouroux, N., Vella, F., Teutsch, P. (2018). Adaptation of user-centered design approaches to abilities of people with disabilities. *ICCHP 2018: Computers Helping People with Special Needs – 16th International Conference*, LNCS, Springer, Cham.

Hassenzahl, M. and Tractinsky, N. (2006). User experience – A research agenda. *Behavior & Information Technology*, 25, 91–97.

Idoughi, D., Seffah, A., Kolski, C. (2012). Adding user experience into the interactive service design loop: A persona-based approach. *Behaviour & Information Technology*, 31(3), 287–303.

Interaction Design Foundation (n.d). Design thinking. *Interaction Design Foundation* [Online]. Available at: https://www.interaction-design.org/literature/topics/design-thinking.

ISO (1998). Ergonomic requirements for office work with visual display terminals – Part 11: Guidance on usability. ISO 9241-11:1998 standard, ISO, Geneva.

ISO (2019). Ergonomie de l'interaction homme-système – Partie 210 : conception centrée sur l'opérateur humain pour les systèmes interactifs. ISO 9241-210:2019 standard, ISO Geneva.

Kensing, F. (2003). *Methods and Practices in Participatory Design*. ITU Press, Copenhagen.

KLAP (2016). Quelles sont les étapes du Design Thinking ? *klap.io* [Online]. Available at: http://www.klap.io/etapes-design-thinking/.

Komminos, A. (2019). 7 UX Deliverables: What will I be making as a UX designer? *Interaction Design Foundation* [Online]. Available at: https://www.interaction-design.org/literature/article/7-ux-deliverables-what-will-i-be-making-as-a-ux-designer.

Krause, R. (2018). Storyboards help visualize UX ideas. *Nielsen Norman Group* [Online]. Available at: https://www.nngroup.com/articles/storyboards-visualize-ideas/.

Lallemand, C. and Gronier, G. (2018). *Méthodes de design UX : 30 méthodes fondamentales pour concevoir et évaluer les systèmes interactifs*. Editions Eyrolles, Paris.

Lee, J.H., Kim, M.J., Kim, S.W. (2015). A study customer journey map for user experience analysis of information and communications technology service. In *DUXU 2015, Part II*, Marcus, A. (ed.). LNCS, Springer. Cham.

Norman, D.A. (1986). Cognitive engineering. In *User Centred System Design: New Perspectives on Human Computer Interaction*, Norman, D.A. and Draper, S.W (eds). Erlbaum, Hillsdale.

Norman, D.A. (2013). *The Design of Everyday Things: Revised and Expanded Edition*. Basic Books, New York.

Sauzin, D. (2017). Apport d'une conception centrée utilisateur adaptée selon les besoins des personnes en situation de handicap. Computer Science PhD Thesis, Université de Toulouse 3, Toulouse.

Schuler, D. and Namioka, A. (1993). *Participatory Design: Principles and Practices.* Erlbaum, Hillsdale.

Seffah, A., Kolski, C., Idoughi, I. (2009). Persona comme outil de design de services interactifs : principes et exemple en e-maintenance. In *Proceedings of the 21st International Conference on Association Francophone d'interaction Homme-Machine IHM '09*, Association for Computing Machinery, New York.

Shostack, G.L. (1977). Breaking free from product marketing. *Journal of Marketing*, 41(2), 73–80.

Stephanidis, C. (2001). *User Interfaces for All: Concepts, Methods and Tools*. CRC Press, Boca Raton.

Stephanidis, C. and Salvendy, G. (1998). Toward an information society for all: An international research and development agenda. *International Journal of Human-Computer Interaction*, 10(2), 107–134.

Touloum, K. (2019). Design de services à partir d'une description des expériences de l'usager : formalisation et application à la gestion de crises. PhD Thesis, University Abderrahmane Mira of Béjaïa, Béjaïa.

Touloum, K., Idoughi, D., Seffah, A. (2012). User eXperience in service design: Defining a common ground from different fields. *4th International Conference on Applied Human Factors and Ergonomics (AHFE)*, San Francisco, 21–25 July.

Touloum, K., Idoughi, D., Seffah, A. (2018). Adding UX in the service design loop: The case of crisis management services. *Interaction Design and Architecture(s) Journal – IxD&A*, 37, 47–77.

UAAG (n.d). User Agent Accessibility Guidelines (UAAG) overview [Online]. Available at: https://www.w3.org/WAI/standards-guidelines/uaag/.

W3C (2017). How people with disabilities use the Web. *Web Accessibility Initiative* [Online]. Available at: https://www.w3.org/WAI/people-use-web/tools-techniques/.

WAI (n.d). Making the Web accessible. *Web Accessibility Initiative* [Online]. Available at: https://www.w3.org/WAI/.

WCAG (n.d). Web Content Accessibility Guidelines (WCAG) 2.0 [Online]. Available at: https://www.w3.org/Translations/WCAG20-fr/.

Winance, M. (2008). La notion de handicap et ses transformations à travers les classifications internationales du handicap de l'OMS, 1980 and 2001. *Dynamis*, 28, 377–406.

PART 3

Change Management and Organizational Innovations

Summary of Contributions – Part 3

Jointly Improving the Experience of All Stakeholders in Hospital 4.0: The ICSSURP Initiative, *by Wilson GOUDALO, Christophe KOLSKI and Frédéric VANDERHAEGEN*

In a rapidly evolving world, we are currently witnessing the inauguration of digital technologies, as seen through the growing importance of new concepts and fields: Cloud Computing, Block Chain, Big Data, Artificial Intelligence, Machine Learning & Deep Learning. The hospital is no exception to this trend and is experiencing a transformation towards Hospital 4.0 (also called the "Hospital of the Future" or "Smart Hospital"). Accordingly, this transformation increasingly allows hospitals to acquire these smart and connected components in different aspects of their value chains; on the one hand, to improve the quality of healthcare at an optimized cost, and, on the other hand, to meet the expectations and objectives of different stakeholders. In this chapter, the authors present the context typical of the digital transformation to Hospital 4.0, and the qualities of Hospital Information Systems 4.0 (HIS 4.0) essential to this process: from security, usability, resilience and performance to the introduction of initiatives such as Joint Security, Safety, Usability, Resilience and Performance Engineering ("*Ingénierie Conjointe de la Sécurité, de la Sûreté, de l'Utilisabilité, de la Résilience et de la Performance*" or *"ICSSURP"*).

Tool-based Approach to Analyze Operating Room Schedule Execution: Application to Online Management, *by Leah RIFI, Franck FONTANILI and Michel JEANNEY*

The operating theater is one of the hospital's most important services, which explains the necessity to make it profitable. This contribution concerns the operating rooms of the *Narbonne Hospital Center, France (NHC)*. The study focuses on *online management*, a function generally performed by an experienced paramedical or medical officer. The research question that the authors try to answer is the following: How do we assist online management to reduce deviations between the initial schedule and the performed schedule, in order to maintain the OR activity at the targeted performance level? To achieve this, they propose a tool-based approach for retrospective analysis of the daily execution of the OR schedule. This punctual analysis is part of a more global approach for continuous improvement in the management of the activity. An example of its applicability is presented through a real-world practical carried out at the *NHC*.

Planning Patient Journeys in Outpatient Hospitals to Support the Ambulatory Shift, *by Virginie FORTINEAU and Lucie ROUSSEL*

The development of outpatient medicine is an important organizational issue for public hospitals that have not been sufficiently configured for the intense nature of "same-day" healthcare. This contribution therefore focuses on the development of outpatient medicine, through dedicated clinics and support for institutions with regard to the ambulatory shift. The authors propose macro-planning for groups of pathways with a Sales and Operation Plan (S&Op), in order to help institutions correctly measure their resources and plan patient pathways. This method has been applied to three real-world examples. The limitations and prospects of this methodology for outpatient medical structures are discussed at the end of the chapter.

Treatment Protocols Generated by Machine Learning: Putting a Case Study of Hospitalization at Home into Perspective, *by Alice MARTIN, Jean-Baptiste GUILLAUME, Alain GUINET and Julien FONDREVELLE*

Hospitalization at home (HaH) is an alternative to traditional hospitalization. It enables a range of medical and paramedical healthcare to be performed in the patient's home, thereby offering them quality and continual healthcare in a familiar living environment. This alternative is gaining popularity since it allows traditional hospitals to focus on healthcare missions that require significant medico-technical resources by shortening or avoiding hospitalization. HaH covers a range of technical and complex healthcare services, which makes it a solution that is particularly suited to vulnerable populations of all ages, who suffer from heavy, progressive, chronic and/or unstable polypathologies. This chapter looks at the various setups and attempts to address the following issues: What are the organizational challenges of HaHs today? How can protocolization respond to them and within what limits? How can the forecast of the trajectory and the cost of the patient stay automatically generate protocols?

Resilience of Healthcare Teams: Case Study of Two Cardiology Intensive Care Units, *by Racha LAMARI*

Healthcare organizations are systems open to their environment, which makes them particularly sensitive to external influences. They operate in an uncertain, complex and increasingly restrictive environment. It is for this reason that resilience is omnipresent in medical practice, and is therefore considered as a core element of clinical practice. Studies on resilience in the workplace have mainly focused on resilience at the individual level. However, in healthcare organizations, individuals do not work in a vacuum; this level of analysis is therefore insufficient to capture the complexity of interactions and interdependencies and understand the processes at stake within the team, which contribute to the risk management of uncertain events. This contribution explores knowledge about how team resilience is developed and deployed. It identifies the resources that make a team resilient, and also explores the activities that the resources can be invested in.

11

Jointly Improving the Experience of All Stakeholders in Hospital 4.0: The ICSSURP Initiative

11.1. Introduction

In a rapidly evolving world, we are currently witnessing the inauguration of new connected, digital technologies. This is evident by the growing importance placed on emergent concepts and fields, including: Cloud Computing, Block Chain, Big Data, Artificial Intelligence, Machine Learning and Deep Learning. These are being exploited or adapted for entertainment purposes, but for essential services and operations of vital importance as well. Therefore, advances in Artificial Intelligence (for further reading on this subject, we recommend Marquis *et al.* 2020a, 2020b, 2020c) and Self-Learning Systems, which exploit Machine Learning and Deep Learning methods (Goodfellow *et al.* 2016), are progressively being amalgamated into components such as software, applications, devices, facilities and even "appliances", which permit it to connect to networks (Ronte *et al.* 2018). These components are often referred to as "smart components" and are increasingly being integrated into all spheres of activity, thanks to easier connectivity, higher computing power, on-demand processing, and the capacity to take advantage of very large volumes of heterogeneous data.

Hospital 4.0 (also called the Hospital of the Future, Intelligent Hospital, Smart Hospital and H.40) is increasingly equipped with these intelligent and connected components for different aspects of its value chain, relating to supply, production, distribution and the entire business model (Frisch 2014, Maddux 2019). Hospital 4.0 is patient-centered and strives to put the patient at the heart of all of its activities and

Chapter written by Wilson GOUDALO, Christophe KOLSKI and Frédéric VANDERHAEGEN.

concerns (Anhang Price *et al.* 2014; Sebastian 2019). Nevertheless, Hospital 4.0 also needs to comply with legal and regulatory requirements, respect its commitments to its stakeholders and meet their respective objectives (Health Quality Ontario 2019). Some of these objectives may seem more difficult to reconcile than others, and at the same time, the hospital is at risk of becoming a playground for cybercrime and geopolitical rivalries (Cerulus 2020).

In the rest of this chapter, we present the context of the digital transformation to Hospital 4.0, followed by the essential qualities of ISH 4.0 as seen through the perspectives on security, usability, resilience and performance engineering by way of introducing our ICSSURP initiative, *Ingénierie Conjointe de la Sécurité, de la Sûreté, de l'Utilisabilité, de la Résilience et de la Performance* (the "Joint Security, Safety, Usability, Resilience and Performance Engineering" initiative).

11.2. Digital transformation to Hospital 4.0

Starting from Web 1.0 (1993–2000) to Web 4.0 (2012–2020), we have moved from the Internet of Content, to the Internet of Communications, to the Internet of Contexts, to the Internet of Things (Lampropoulos *et al.* 2019). Objects are increasingly endowed with intelligence (in the sense of Artificial Intelligence – AI), and can communicate with each other, with traditional information systems and in a targeted (personalized) manner with individuals or groups of people (Bozic 2019).

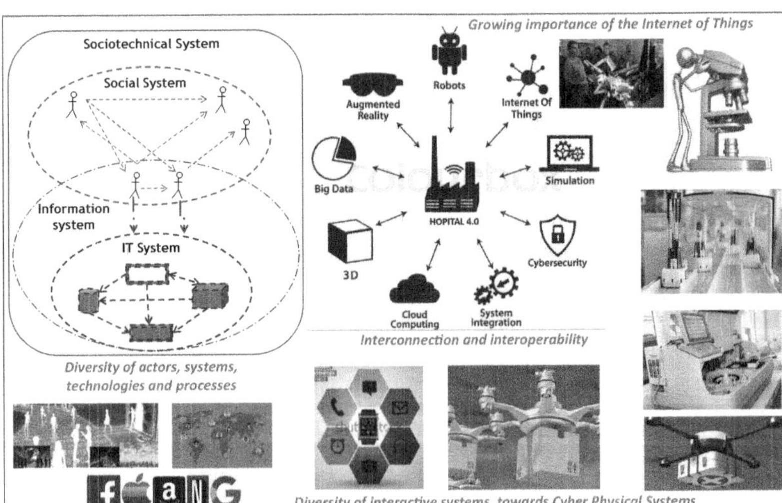

Figure 11.1. *The modern-day digital context of Hospital 4.0. For a color version of this figure, see www.iste.co.uk/chaabane/healthcare.zip*

In the socio-technical context of Hospital 4.0 (see Figure 11.1), Cyber Physical Systems (CPS) interact with humans on aspects of health and vital interventions (ANSSI 2020). The digital transformation of Hospital 4.0 presents very significant challenges (Circle Square 2019). In addition to the context of socio-technical systems (Coakes 2002; Singh 2013), Hospital 4.0 is made up of a wide variety of connected objects and a large number of heterogeneous platforms that must interact for a high-quality health service. The challenges facing Hospital 4.0 pertain to: interoperability between devices, technologies and heterogeneous ecosystems; the quality of the data processed and returned, which in turn must be precise and reliable; the reliability for services of vital importance; the continuity of trustworthy operations and services; the guarantee of data and processing security; the requirements to respect privacy and the protection of personal information and health data; compliance with legal and regulatory requirements; easy collaboration between several stakeholders; advanced and intelligent analysis of data and services (Big Data Analytics); the guarantee of engaging, optimized and personalized health services that take into account the cultural and socioeconomic context.

These challenges, inestimable but pertinent, can be classified and prioritized according to different perspectives and objectives. They present obstacles that are both scientific (due to their intercorrelations, there is often need for tough trade-offs) and technical (involving very dynamic technological innovations). As discussed in the outlook, we plan to classify this according to business systems and investment management approaches. This classification must therefore take into account, among other things, technological criteria, criteria for regulatory and legal compliance, criteria for human and societal values, sustainability criteria and economic criteria.

11.3. Essential qualities of information systems of Hospital 4.0

A successful interoperability should make interactions more fluid and facilitate collaboration and cooperation between healthcare professionals, healthcare specialists and patients, in order to make the most accurate diagnoses and provide the best healthcare, suited to each patient and at an optimized cost, in compliance with regulatory and legal constraints. Thanks to artificial intelligence, self-learning systems and connected objects, patients can progressively play a more prominent role in Hospital 4.0, with their feedback, experience and feelings being considered differently. Ultimately, the diagnoses will be made earlier, with better precision and greater anticipation, to the greatest extent possible. Prescriptions and interventions could eventually become more insightful and more appropriate for each patient in terms of their cultural and socio-technical context.

All Information Systems of Hospital 4.0 (ISH 4.0) require appropriate features (qualities), characterized by qualitative and quantitative criteria that must be defined and managed harmoniously at all levels. The processing of sensitive data and the provision of services of vital importance requires ISH 4.0 to have increased information security (ANSSI 2020). The provision of services and products that are used and consumed by humans also requires ISH 4.0 to have quality human–computer interactions (HCI), in particular, effective usability. Contributing primarily to operations and interventions of vital importance, ISH 4.0 must have good resilience, particularly in the event of incidents, accidents or crisis situations. Operated by several stakeholders and actors in socio-economic and cultural life, ISH 4.0 also need to have good performance (Health Quality Ontario 2019).

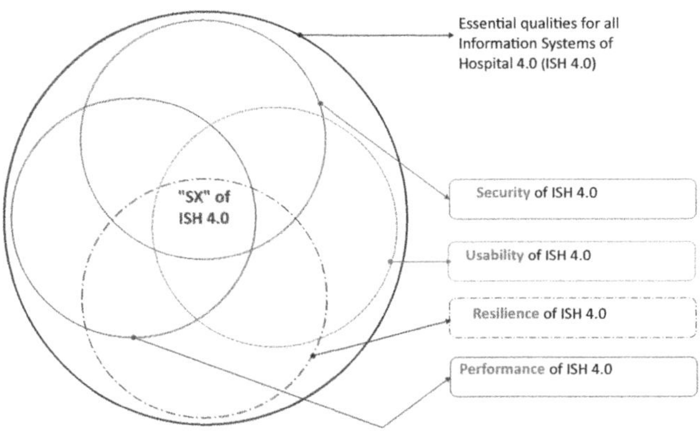

Figure 11.2. *Information systems of Hospital 4.0 (ISH4.0) and their essential qualities ISH 4.0. For a color version of this figure, see www.iste.co.uk/chaabane/healthcare.zip*

11.3.1. *Security in information systems of Hospital 4.0*

In all security standards (local and international), the three invariant criteria are the same: Confidentiality, Integrity and Availability (ISO 2010; ANSSI 2020; NIST 2020). Further to these three fundamental criteria, several features (qualities) and security properties are added, such as proof, tracing, non-repudiation, identification and authentication, which have been combined to establish the concept of accountability. In the Information Systems of Hospital 4.0, the qualities of respect for privacy and trust are explicitly linked to security.

An incident that can result in the loss of accountability, confidentiality, integrity or availability can cause potentially significant impact to systems (Gonzales *et al.* 2020), as shown in Table 11.1. In the digital services industry, incidents are linked to three concepts: technical problems, security attacks and errors (relating to the human factor). In ISH 4.0, the threats to each of these three incident concepts can become greater in magnitude: (1) the very high risk of technical problems (due to the complexity of interconnections, equipment and devices; the plurality and heterogeneity of applications and services from different sources; the orchestration of business with disparate activities, national and cross-border organizations, in the face of increased socio-economic and geopolitical impacts); (2) the sophistication of security attacks (very strong motivations and high interests for well-qualified individuals and for well-organized groups that commit high-intensity attacks and abuse of all kinds in order to achieve their objectives, the availability of significant resources and kits for hackers and cyber attackers, a well-justified desire to "open up" the different systems); and (3) higher risks involving human factors and associated errors (information technology consumerism, emergence of ubiquitous systems, BYOD – Bring Your Own Device, increased demand for immediacy, greater consumptive dependence on digital services in personal, social, administrative and professional activities, the gradual disappearance of barriers between social networks, private systems and corporate networks). With a view to managing all types of incidents, we propose the ICSSURP initiative, outlined in section 11.4, for advanced security engineering that encompasses the usability, resilience and performance of ISH 4.0.

Protection Objectives	Potential Impacts
Accountability	Losses in traceability, audit trails and transparency. Loss of brand image and penalties for regulatory non-compliance.
Availability	Direct operation losses and loss of market share.
Confidentiality	Disclosure of sensitive information, penalties for non-compliance, loss of reputation and market share.
Integrity	Data corruption, service inconsistency, loss of reputation and market share.

Table 11.1. *Security impacts*

11.3.2. *Usability of information systems of Hospital 4.0*

Usability is a very rich and well-studied criterion (Nielsen 1994; Lewis 2014). The guarantee of usability allows users to achieve their goals and meet their needs within a particular context of use. The context of use takes into account users, tasks, equipment, and physical and social environments, which can all influence the usability of a service (product or system).

The ISO 9241-11 standard describes the usability measure in terms of user performance and user satisfaction (ISO 2018). It specifies that the measure for performance and user satisfaction needs to take into account: the ways in which the initial planned usage of objectives is achieved; the nature and quantity of resources that must be deployed in order to achieve the objective targets; and how the user finds the use of the product or service satisfactory. Usable products and services can be designed by directly incorporating the known features that benefit users in particular contexts of use into their specifications (characteristics). Shackel (2009) assesses usability based on three criteria: performance in completing the task, user satisfaction and cost. Usability performance breaks down into effectiveness and efficiency. Usability engineering refers to a design process that addresses, qualitatively, quantitatively and predictively, the usability of a product, system or service. In order to specify or measure usability, the ISO 9241-11 standard recommends identifying the objectives and breaking down effectiveness, efficiency, satisfaction and components within the context of use into sub-components, with qualities that are measurable and demonstrable.

Table 11.2 presents a summary of the usability objectives and the associated potential risks.

Usability Objectives	Potential Impacts
Cost of use (in carrying out a task)	Source of errors
Efficiency of task completion	Source of workaround and/or abandonment
Efficiency of task performance	Source of errors and/or security breaches
User satisfaction in carrying out tasks	Source of rejection and/or workaround

Table 11.2. *Usability impacts*

11.3.3. *Resilience of information systems of Hospital 4.0*

According to social psychology, in industry or in business, the notion of resilience presents the capacity for "bouncing back" from an incident, whatever the nature of it (Engle *et al.* 1996; Hamel and Välikangas 2003; Hollnagel *et al.* 2006). The notion of an incident relating to resilience represents concepts such as: adversity, changes in risk, forces of circumstance. Based on the work of Laprie and Luzeaux (Laprie 2008; Luzeaux 2011), we define resilience as a dynamic process conferring the capacity to provide justifiable trust for services, on the one hand, by avoiding too frequent or too severe failures, and, on the other hand, by ensuring the persistence of reliable service delivery, even in the event of any type of incident. Resilience can be seen as a system's capacity to control, succeed and adapt to disturbances within (Cuvelier 2013; Vanderhaegen 2017). Resilience relates to the ability of a system, or a human being, to avoid any loss of self-control, or to maintain self-control despite the occurrence of disturbances (Vanderhaegen 2016,

2017, 2021). Resilience engineering states that variability is not only normal, but necessary for the proper functioning and success of a system. Note that in this regard, resilience is considered essential for long-term systems (Ruault 2015).

Resilience is the capacity of a socio-technical system to continue to fulfill its operational mission and avoid unacceptable consequences, despite diverse disturbances (exceptional constraints, difficult conditions, unforeseen events). This definition takes into account response time, cost of recovery and severity of damage. In most cases, there are three main sources of incidents that can cause disruption to a socio-technical system (technical problem, human error, attack or embezzlement). Resilience techniques anticipate, treat and limit the severity of the consequences from conceivable disturbances. In addition to security and usability solutions, in the event of risk occurrences, resilience makes it possible to tolerate and exceed these impacts, and is able to guarantee degraded services in accordance with the conditions of the service level agreement (SLA), with respect to user experience (Goudalo 2017). Table 11.3 presents resilience techniques with regard to resilience objectives.

Resilience Objectives	Resilience Techniques
Avoid unacceptable incidents, in terms of frequency and severity, in the event of a change	Scalability (adaptability)
Guarantee the continued provision of trust services	Assessment and verification
Take into account system changes	Usability for both human and non-human users (of applications, services and systems)
Take into account the complexity of systems	Diversity (increasing the diversity of means and take advantage of alternative means in order to avoid SPOF – Single Point Of Failure (Dooley 2001))

Table 11.3. *Resilience techniques*

11.3.4. *Performance of information systems of Hospital 4.0*

The performance of ISH 4.0 is a field in its own right, which will undoubtedly become a source for changes in the years to come (Routelous 2013; Thibodeau 2018; Health Quality Ontario 2019). Here, performance can be defined from the point of view of the business of Hospital 4.0 in terms of patients (their real earnings and contributions), doctors and practitioners (that which they devote themselves, body and soul, to), investors (their expectations), public powers (demands on health systems), directors, managers and staff (their daily battles).

We have dealt with the essential qualities of ISH 4.0 through the lenses of security, usability, resilience and performance, and their reciprocal correlations, collectively. Figure 11.2 illustrates the positioning of the Stakeholder eXperience (SX) involved, through the collective and harmonious management of the four axes that define the essential qualities of Information Systems of Hospital 4.0 ("SX" of ISH 4.0).

11.4. Towards a joint security, safety, usability, resilience and performance engineering initiative (ICSSURP)

For the ICSSURP initiative (the "Joint Security, Safety, Usability, Resilience and Performance" initiative) of Hospital 4.0, we propose an advanced conceptual model and a homogeneous metric system.

11.4.1. *Advanced conceptual model of ICSSURP*

Figure 11.3 presents the advanced conceptual model of the ICSSURP initiative, inspired by Goudalo *et al.* (2017b). Our advanced conceptual model aims to jointly model security, resilience, usability and performance, with the goal of improving the user experience of all of the stakeholders in Hospital 4.0. The advanced conceptual model collectively operates on assets, incident risks and solutions. It must be able to be supported by a homogeneous metric system that also operates on these three axes.

11.4.2. *System of homogeneous metrics*

By drawing inspiration from the deliberations outlined in Goudalo (2017), a homogeneous metric system has to be proposed. The one proposed in this chapter could be graded "0", "1", "2" and "3" for each of the three axes corresponding to assets, risk of incidents and solutions. Well-defined metrics promote communication with stakeholders in order to take into account everyone's concerns. Our joint engineering operates on concepts that are measured and evaluated quantitatively and qualitatively within a metric system, in order to guarantee proper management. We offer four types of measures: Technical (related to technologies and business processes), Organizational, Costs and Satisfaction. We express the values associated with metrics in quantitative, qualitative or semi-quantitative terms.

In the case of assets, we have developed metrics as Cartesian products of qualities and values, such as pairs (quality, value). We have defined the qualities of each of the four domains (security, usability, resilience and performance) and where they intersect. The qualities identified are the 14 criteria shown in Figure 11.3:

Accountability, Availability, Confidentiality, Compliance, Cost, Effectiveness, Substantial Value (SV), Efficiency, Integrity, Maintainability, Reliability, Security, Satisfaction, Tolerance Level of Harm (TLH).

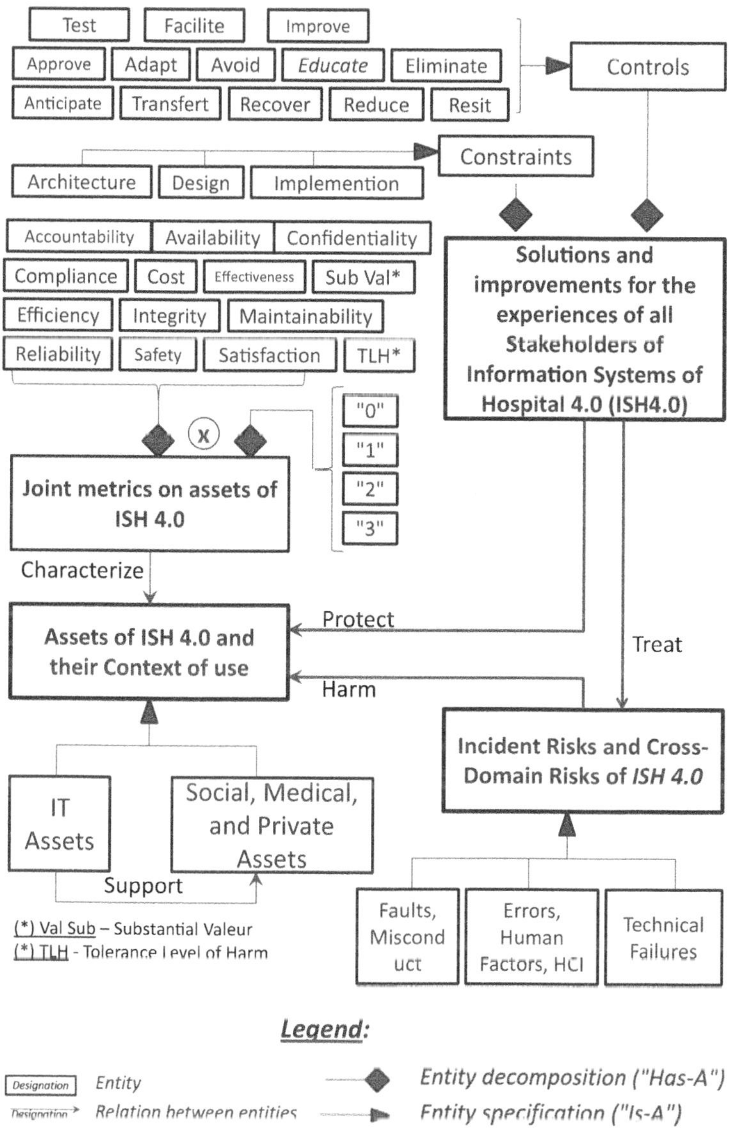

Figure 11.3. *Information systems of Hospital 4.0 and the advanced conceptual model of the ICSSURP initiative. For a color version of this figure, see www.iste.co.uk/chaabane/healthcare.zip*

For reasons of homogeneity, efficiency and ease of handling, we propose to standardize values into four categories: “Not applicable or Very Low – 0”, “Low – 1”, “High – 2” and “Very high – 3”. Concerning the risk of incidents, we propose to standardize the metrics into four levels, in relation to the probability of occurrence, exposure surface and severity. Likewise, these four levels of risk of incidents are as follows: “Not applicable or Very Low – 0”, “Low – 1”, “High – 2” and “Very high – 3”. As for the solutions, we offer four standardized levels that define their effectiveness, according to the levels of risk of incidents and actions on the assets involved. Whether the solutions are controls and/or constraints, the four standardized solution levels remain the same: “Not applicable or Very Low – 0”, “Ineffective – 1”, “Effective – 2” and “Very effective – 3”.

11.4.3. *Summary of the ICSSURP initiative*

Based on this advanced conceptual model, the ICSSURP initiative defines a holistic approach for developing Joint Safety, Security, Usability, Resilience and Performance. The criteria relating to Performance, Resilience, Security and Usability, with their respective values, characterize the assets of the Information Systems of Hospital 4.0, which are threatened by the risks typical to ISH 4.0. Appropriate solutions, composed of controls and constraints, with improved experience for all stakeholders, will address the risks and protect ISH 4.0 (Information Systems of Hospital 4.0) assets in their contexts of use.

Security leads to a different consideration of health personnel, in particular doctors, surgeons, anesthesiologists, caregivers, and in certain cases, patients as well; for further reading on this subject, the potential diversity of actors in healthcare who are users of medical devices, see the study by Shah and Robinson (2008). In addition to medical devices currently in use, they will need to use devices that are connected to ISH 4.0. Death or the risk of worsening health conditions, serious infections or improper care due to human error could be considered as part of the improved reliability that Hospital 4.0 will provide. As such, we are able to refocus on the ICSSURP initiative, which will aim to facilitate the establishment and adoption of Hospital 4.0 by guaranteeing its promises, improving the situation of staff and providing better patient care at optimized costs.

11.5. Conclusion and perspectives

In the next iteration, the aim will be to work more closely with researchers and specialists in the hospital and healthcare industry, in order to propose, on the one hand, an enterprise architecture which will have to support the digital transformation to Hospital 4.0, and, on the other hand, a formalization of the vocabulary used by notation diagrams, such as an extension of UML or SysML. These two new contributions will lead to the substantial development of the ICSSURP initiative, which will outline the framework for the next three components that we are considering.

Given the criticality of the hospital as an operator of vital importance, and that Hospital 4.0 will increase this criticality, we are aiming to refocus the first part of our work on advanced resilience engineering approaches. A resilient ISH 4.0 (Information Systems of Hospital 4.0) will firstly have to prevent, absorb, recover or mitigate against any problem, secondly, it will have to successfully control unprecedented situations, thirdly, it will have to successfully self-organize the components of the interconnected system to react to any failure, and fourthly, it will also have to integrate the principle of human-systems inclusion, in order to optimize online and offline learning processes, involving technical and human systems. The second part of our work will aim to classify the plethora of challenges facing ISH 4.0, according to business systems and investment management approaches. Finally, the third component will focus on approaches to optimize Business Process Management (BPM) initiatives and activities, giving ISH 4.0 the ability to sufficiently contribute to meeting new performance requirements being placed on the hospital, and in addition, those yet to be placed on Hospital 4.0.

This chapter presented the digital context of Hospital 4.0 and the challenges and issues it faces. The interests and feasibility of a joint and harmonious approach were presented, not only for better patient care, but also for the better health and well-being of our populations. The GISEH conferences could represent a scientific opportunity to assist in the steady development of the ICSSURP initiative. Several themes and areas for development for the ICSSURP initiative have been presented above. Several other enriching directions could be identified through contact with experts and professionals in the field, as well as through contact with patients and other stakeholders of Hospital 4.0.

11.6. References

Anhang Price, R., Elliott, M.N., Zaslavsky, A.M., Hays, R.D., Lehrman, W.G., Rybowski, L., Edgman-Levitan, S., Cleary, P.D. (2014). Examining the role of patient experience surveys in measuring health care quality. *Medical Care Research and Review*, 71(5), 522–554.

ANSSI (2020). Protection des OIV (Opérateurs d'Importance Vitale) en France [Online]. Available at: https://www.ssi.gouv.fr/ [Accessed October 2020].

Bozic, V. (2019). Smart hospital – Our experience. *Smart Cities and Regional Development (SCRD) Journal*, 3(2), 95–99.

Cerulus, L. (2020). European commission president Ursula von der Leyen called out. *Politico* [Online]. Available at: https://www.politico.eu/ [Accessed October 2020].

Circle Square Inc. (2019). Digital health trends (December 2019) year in review [Online]. Available at: https://www.circlesquareinc.com/trends [Accessed October 2020].

Coakes, E. (2002). Knowledge management: A sociotechnical perspective. In *Knowledge Management in the Sociotechnical World*, Cokes, E., Willis, D., Clarke, S. (eds). Springer-Verlag, London.

Cuvelier, L. (2013). L'ingénierie de la résilience : un nouveau modèle pour améliorer la sécurité des patients ? L'exemple de l'anesthésie. *Santé Publique*, 25, 475–482.

Dooley, K. (2001). *Designing Large Scale LANs*. O'Reilly Media, Inc, Sebastopol, CA.

Engle, P.L., Castle, S., Menon, P. (1996). Child development: Vulnerability and resilience. *Social Science and Medicine*, 43(5), 621–635.

Frisch, P. (2014). What is an intelligent hospital? A place where technology and design converge to enhance patient care. *IEEE Pulse*, 5(6), 10–15.

Gonzales, D., Harting, S., Adgie, M.K., Brackup, J., Stanley, K.D. (2020). Unclassified and secure: A defense industrial base cyber protection program for unclassified defense networks. *RAND Corporation* [Online]. Available at: https://www.rand.org/pubs/research_reports/RR4227.html [Accessed October 2020].

Goodfellow, I.J., Bengio, Y., Courville, A. (2016). *Deep Learning*. MIT Press, Cambridge, MA.

Goudalo, W. (2017). Vers une ingénierie avancée de la sécurité des systèmes d'information d'entreprise : une approche conjointe de la sécurité, de l'utilisabilité et de la résilience dans les systèmes sociotechniques. PhD Thesis, Université de Valenciennes et du Hainaut-Cambrésis, Valenciennes.

Goudalo, W., Kolski, C., Vanderhaegen, F. (2017a). Towards advanced security engineering for enterprise information systems: Solving security, resilience and usability issues together within improvement of user experience. International Conference on *Enterprise Information Systems*, LNCS, Springer, 291, 436–459.

Goudalo, W., Kolski, C., Vanderhaegen, F. (2017b). Vers une ingénierie avancée de la sécurité des SI d'entreprise : une approche conjointe de la sécurité, de l'utilisabilité et de la résilience dans les systèmes sociotechniques. *Ingénierie des Systèmes d'Information*, 22(1), 65–107.

Hamel, G. and Välikangas, L. (2003). The quest for resilience. *Harvard Business Review*, Brighton, MA.

Health Quality Ontario (2019). The performance of Ontario's health system: Measuring up 2019 [Online]. Available at: https://www.hqontario.ca/System-Performance/Yearly-Reports/Measuring-Up-2019 [Accessed October 2020].

Hollnagel, E., Woods, D., Leveson, N. (2006). *Resilience Engineering: Concepts and Precepts*. Ashgate Publishing, Aldershot.

ISO (2018). ISO 9241-11:2018. Ergonomie de l'interaction homme-système – Partie 11 : Utilisabilité – Définitions et concepts.

ISO/IEC (2010). ISO/IEC 27000. Information technology – Security techniques.

ISO/IEC (2012). ISO/IEC 27032. Information technology – Security techniques – Guidelines for security.

Lampropoulos, G., Siakas, K., Anastasiadis, T. (2019). Internet of things in the context of industry 4.0: An overview. *International Journal of Entrepreneurial Knowledge*, 7(1), 4–19.

Laprie, J.C. (2008). About resilience – From dependability to resilience. *IFIP Working Group 10.4 on Dependable Computing and Fault Tolerance*, 54th meeting. Alyeska, AK.

Lewis, J.R. (2014). Usability: Lessons learned… and yet to be learned. *International Journal of Human-Computer Interaction*, 30(9), 663–684.

Luzeaux, D. (2011). Engineering large-scale complex systems. In *Complex Systems and Systems of Systems Engineering*, Luzeaux, D., Ruault J.-R., Wippler, J.-L. (eds). ISTE Ltd, London, and John Wiley & Sons, New York.

Maddux, F.W. (2019). Transforming healthcare through interconnected intelligence. Global Annual Medical Report for Fresenius Medical Care [Online]. Available at: https://fmcna.com/ [Accessed October 2020].

Marquis, P., Papini, O., Prade, H. (eds) (2020a). *A Guided Tour of Artificial Intelligence Research. Volume I: Knowledge Representation, Reasoning and Learning*. Springer, Cham.

Marquis, P., Papini, O., Prade, H. (eds) (2020b). *A Guided Tour of Artificial Intelligence Research. Volume II: AI Algorithms*. Springer, Cham.

Marquis, P., Papini, O., Prade, H. (eds) (2020c). *A Guided Tour of Artificial Intelligence Research. Volume III: Interfaces and Applications of Artificial Intelligence.* Springer, Cham.

Nielsen, J. (1994). *Usability Engineering*. Morgan Kaufmann Publishers, Burlington, MA.

NIST (2020). Cybersecurity framework [Online]. Available at: https://www.nist.gov/cyberframework [Accessed October 2020].

Ronte, H., Taylor, K., Haughey, J. (2018). Medtech and the internet of medical things: How connected medical devices are transforming health care. Professional report, Deloitte [Online]. Available at: https://www2.deloitte.com [Accessed October 2020].

Routelous, C. (2013). L'hôpital à l'épreuve de la performance économique : doctrines, instruments et hybridations des valeurs. *Quaderni*, 82, 5–16 [Online]. Available at: https://doi.org/10.4000/quaderni.735 [Accessed October 2020].

Ruault, J.R. (2015). Proposition d'architecture et de processus pour la résilience des systèmes ; application aux systèmes critiques à longue durée de vie. Automation PhD Thesis, LAMIH, UVHC, Valenciennes.

Sebastian, M.P. (2019). Smart hospitals: Challenges and opportunities. No. 315, Working papers, Indian Institute of Management, Kozhikode.

Shackel, B. (2009). Usability–context, framework, definition, design, and evaluation. In *Human Factors for Informatics Usability*, Shackel, B. and Richardson S. (eds). Cambridge University Press, Cambridge.

Shah, S.G.S. and Robinson, I. (2008). Medical device technologies: Who is the user? *International Journal of Healthcare Technology and Management*, 9(2), 181–197.

Singh, M.P. (2013). Norms as a basis for governing sociotechnical systems. *ACM Transactions on Intelligent Systems and Technology (TIST)*, 5(1), 1–23, New York.

Thibodeau, Y. (2018). Comment optimiser la performance des hôpitaux ? *PetalMD* [Online]. Available at: https://blog.petal-health.com/fr-ca/comment-optimiser-performance-hopitaux [Accessed October 2020].

Vanderhaegen, F. (2016). A rule-based support system for dissonance discovery and control applied to car driving. *Expert Systems with Applications*, 65, 361–371.

Vanderhaegen, F. (2017). Towards increased systems resilience: New challenges based on dissonance control for human reliability in Cyber-Physical & Human Systems. *Annual Reviews in Control*, 44, 316–322.

Vanderhaegen, F. (2021). Pedagogical learning supports based on human–systems inclusion applied to rail flow control. *Cognition Technology & Work*, 23, 193–202.

12

A Tool-based Approach to Analyze Operating Room Schedule Execution: Application to Online Management

12.1. Introduction

The running costs of an operating suite amount to more than 10% of a hospital's budget, hence the need for its use to be cost-effective (Macario *et al.* 1997). To organize surgical cases as effectively as possible, many studies deal with issues concerning the organization of the operating room (OR) schedule and the mobilization of the resources required.

In this chapter, we define operating room (OR) as the *surgical room* where staff perform surgery on patients, and operating suite as the *surgical department* that houses all the ORs.

The operating suite of the *Centre Hospitalier de Narbonne* (CHN), France, serves as the case study for this chapter. It follows a scheduling strategy called *block scheduling* (Chaabane *et al.* 2007; Koppka *et al.* 2018). It is governed by three decision-making processes which are linked by the following chronology: (1) distribution of allocated OR times (AOT), called shifts, among the different specialties (horizon = 6–12 months); (2) scheduling of the sequence of cases so as to best use AOT, all the while respecting the constraints related to resources (horizon = 1 week); and finally (3) online management, which is at the heart of daily activities management (horizon = 1 day) (ANAP 2016a).

Chapter written by Leah RIFI, Franck FONTANILI and Michel JEANNEY.

This chapter focuses on *online management*, a function generally performed by an experienced paramedic or medical officer. The OR manager is in charge of the smooth execution of the OR schedule by regularly checking the milestones of the patient pathway and minimizing the differences between the *initial schedule* (IS), validated the day before, and the *performed schedule* (PS). These deviations are due to two types of random disruptions: punctual events, which are discrete events affecting schedule execution (e.g. emergency arrival during schedule execution), and uncertainties, which are inaccuracies associated with the estimation of physical measurements (e.g. surgery duration, or the clean-up duration, i.e. the time period following a surgery) (Hammami *et al.* 2007).

There are two operational management approaches to reduce the deviations brought about by disruptions. The first and most common is to integrate random disruptions directly into the IS. In this regard, Aniba and Jebali (2011) and Tancrez *et al.* (2011) propose to include variability into the surgery duration and the emergency case arrivals. The second approach, less documented in the scientific literature, is to make decisions during the execution of the OR schedule. This is essentially the role of online management; a function which is all the more important for activities taking place in a disrupted situation, and which is crucial to the functioning of the operating suite. Unfortunately, it is impossible to prevent disruptions from taking place (Gentil 2013), which is why the remainder of this chapter focuses on online management of disruptions.

The research question we are trying to answer is as follows: How can online management be supported to reduce deviations between the IS and the PS, in order to maintain OR activity at the desired performance level? To achieve this, we propose a tool-based approach for a retrospective analysis of the daily execution of the OR schedule. This punctual analysis is part of a more global approach for the continuous improvement of operational management. The phases are as follows: (1) reconstruct the execution of the OR schedule by highlighting the deviations from the IS and the actions implemented to remedy these; (2) identify, quantify and assess the random daily disruptions as well as their root cause(s); and (3) identify and assess the relevance of the actions and decisions of online management.

In the second section of this chapter, we detail the methodology which allows us, through successive iterations, to generate our tool-based approach. In the third section, we detail the tools upon which it is based. Finally, the last section illustrates its applicability through a concrete example of online management at the *Centre Hospitalier de Narbonne*.

12.2. Methodology used to generate our approach

This section describes the different phases needed to reproduce our tool-based approach. We propose a first version of our approach after a preliminary phase of modeling. Then, thanks to an iterative cycle in three phases, we seek to confirm that our work achieves the objectives initially set.

12.2.1. *Preliminary phase: from observation to the approach outline*

This preliminary phase consists of observing and modeling the operations of the operating suite. It is completed by iterative cycles aimed at designing, building and testing tools. This allows us to define a first draft of our approach and to improve it over successive iterations. We offer two tools. The first is a Dashboard which calculates indicators through quantitative data. These indicators make it possible to assess the quality of the scheduling, to highlight any deviation(s) from the IS and to determine their root cause(s), as well as their impact on the OR schedule. The second is a Logbook, which, on the basis of time-stamped events and qualitative data, lists the disruptions taken into account by the OR manager throughout the day, as well as the decisions taken to integrate these into the schedule, or those taken to anticipate them.

12.2.2. *Phase 1: design*

In this phase, we build and offer conceptual models of the two tools used to collect and structure the data, as well as a description of the different stages of our approach. This phase makes it possible to validate the consistency of our proposals with the requirements and the realties on the ground, before moving forward with their development. The OR manager provides expertise to analyze *a posteriori* the schedule execution while taking into account the reality and complexity of the processes being studied. In the event of a gap between what the tool offers and what is really needed, it may be necessary to return to the preliminary observation phase.

The Dashboard conceptual model lists the indicators that are used to assess the quality of the OR schedule, to compare them, to objectify the deviations and to identify their root cause(s) and impact on the PS. For each indicator, the model describes the necessary initial data, the data collection method (schedule interpretation, data extraction from the OR information system, data extraction for agent's statements, computations, etc.), the scope (operating suite, OR, single deviation), the calculation method (formula) and finally the data interpretation method (performance threshold, target, etc.). An example is shown in Table 12.1. The Logbook conceptual model describes the structure of the entries and suggests data to be collected for each of them. The Logbook conceptual model is detailed in section 12.4. The resulting approach is presented in section 12.3.

Indicator	Late start
Input data (for IS and PS)	T1 = Time of start of shift, T2 = Time of first patient entering the ward, D1 = Allocated OR Time
Data collection method	Interpreting schedules or extracting data from the OR information system
Scope of the indicator	Compute the indicators for each OR and for the entire operating suite
Formula	Late start time = max (T2–T1; 0) Late start rate = max ((T2–T1)/D1; 0)
Interpretation method	Target: 0% ≤ late start rate ≤ 5%

Table 12.1. *Example of a dashboard conceptual model for indicators linked to a late start: duration of late start and the late start rate*

12.2.3. *Phase 2: build*

In this phase, we move on to the actual construction of the tools. In doing so, we check that we can actually build them despite the technical constraints that exist, such as difficulties extracting initial data necessary for the calculation of indicators.

For the Dashboard, the first step is to choose a format that makes it possible to build an intuitive and easy-to-use tool. It can, for example, be a software to process and visualize data like *Excel* or *Power BI*. Next, it is necessary to collect the initial data, compute the new indicators and, if required, correct the previous ones. Finally, we need to create visuals for the indicators (e.g. tables, pie charts, etc.). For the Logbook, we must first choose a format (e.g. Excel spreadsheet, Word document, paper notebook, etc.) that is intuitive and easy to use since the actions of the OR manager can be very close in time and information dense.

12.2.4. *Phase 3: test*

In this phase, we check that the tool-based approach achieves the initial objectives that we have set for ourselves. We propose: (1) to test the tools in order to determine whether the approach allows for the planned analysis; (2) to have the process applied by the agent who will be responsible for it; and (3) to assess the obtained results. We then loop back to Phase 1 (Design) in order to correct any defects uncovered and improve existing functionalities.

12.3. Current version of the proposed tool-based approach

In this section, we present our two tools in detail, as well as the different stages of the proposed approach. The analysis also relies on the interpretation of the IS and PS. This allows us to know the range, the start and the end times of the surgeries and the clean-ups between each intervention.

12.3.1. *Presentation of the first tool: the dashboard conceptual model*

12.3.1.1. *Presentation of our basic dashboard indicators*

The scientific literature is full of sets of indicators dedicated to OR management (Macario 2006; Samudra *et al.* 2016). In order to objectively study this schedule, we use basic indicators as defined and recommended by the ANAP, *L'Agence Nationale de l'Appui à la Performance* (i.e. the National Performance Support Agency for medico-social establishments) (ANAP 2016b). We present these five indicators in Table 12.2. The target indicated is that recommended by (ANAP 2016a). Before the first case of the day, the nurse anesthetists (CRNA: Certified Registered Nurse Anesthetist) must prepare the OR for the patient; this is "the opening of the OR". This process usually takes between 10 and 15 minutes. At the CHN, a late start is inevitable because the CRNA schedule starts at the same time as the AOT. Thus, they do not have enough time to open the OR before the start of the operating day. The time between cases is the sum of the clean-up delays (from when the patient exits the OR to the start of the OR clean-up), and the patient entry delays (from the end of the OR clean-up after a surgery to the entry of the next patient).

We also propose to study Surgical Duration (SD), Clean-up Duration (CUD), Total Case Duration (TCD = SD + CUD) as well as their percentage as compared to the Allocated OR Time. Finally, we calculate the deviations (or differences) for each of these indicators between the IS and the PS. These deviations can be calculated in relation to the IS or in relation to an ideal schedule which respects good scheduling practices and does not contain any inconsistencies (see Table 12.4). For example, during a perfect schedule execution, there is no patient entry delay or early stop.

Indicator	Definition	Target
Utilization rate (UR)	[Utilization time]/AOT	85%
Late start rate (LSR)	[Unused time at the start of the AOT]/AOT	<5%
Early stop rate (ESR)	[Unused time at the end of the AOT]/AOT	<5%
Restricted overtime rate (ROR)	[Sum of the surgery duration outside of the AOT less than an hour after or before the AOT]/AOT *Does not include the last clean-up duration	<5%
Time between cases rate (BCR)	[Unused time between the cases during the AOT]/AOT	<5%

Table 12.2. *Performance indicators and their target values for the operating suite, as proposed by the ANAP*

12.3.1.2. *Calculation of indicators with different scales*

As part of our study, we chose to look at the indicators in the form of ratios – as a percentage of Allocated OR Time – and in the form of durations, i.e. without dividing the numerator by the AOT. We calculated them over a day at different spatial scales: a surgical case, an OR and the operating suite. In this section, we explain the computations for an operating suite and for an OR.

Consider an operating suite with n ORs indexed by $j = \{1; \ldots; n\}$. Consider an OR j which accommodates p_j cases indexed $i = \{1; \ldots; p_j\}$. I_{case}, I_{room} and I_{suite} are the indicators in the form of duration calculated on the three scales mentioned. We show that the indicator is a ratio by adding a "%" symbol after I. The calculation of an indicator for an OR j or for the entire operating suite is presented in equations [12.1] and [12.2], respectively.

$$I\%_{room}(j) = \sum_{i=1}^{p_j} \frac{I_{case}(i,j)}{AOT\ (j)} \qquad [12.1]$$

$$I\%_{suite} = \frac{1}{n}\sum_{j=1}^{n} I\%_{room}(j) = \frac{1}{n}\sum_{i,j} \frac{I_{case}(i,j)}{AOT\ (j)} \qquad [12.2]$$

EXAMPLE.– Take an operating suite with two ORs: OR#1 and OR#2. OR#1 hosts two cases whose Intervention Durations are, respectively, 1.5 h and 1.25 h, and whose Allocated OR Time is 4 h. OR#2's utilization rate is 85%. We seek to calculate the utilization rate of OR#1 and of the entire operating suite. The utilization rate for OR#1 is (1.5 h + 1.25 h)/4 h = 68.75% and the utilization rate of the entire operating suite is (68.75 + 85)/2 = 76.87%.

Note that we add the indicators to go from the scale of a case to that of an OR, and that we take an average to go from an OR to the entire operating suite.

12.3.2. *Presentation of the second tool: the Logbook*

Table 12.3 describes the information to be collected in the Logbook for disruptions (lines 1–5) and the actions implemented to remedy them (lines 6–8).

Inputs	Writing assistance	No.
ID	Unique identifier linked to the disruption	1
H detection	Time of detection by the OR manager	2
Description	It is possible to draw inspiration from the QQOQCCP tool (Pauchard 2010)	3
Impact	Impact of the disruption on the OR schedule in terms of avoidable or unavoidable temporal delays/advances	4
Root causes	Source of disruption. It is possible to draw inspiration from the 5P tool (Pauchard 2010)	5
Time action	Time of OR manager's actions/decisions	6
Description	Options considered, selected and justification for this choice	7
Outcomes	Consequence of this decision/action on the OR schedule. Evaluation *a posteriori* of its relevance	8

Table 12.3. *Description of Logbook entries*

12.3.3. *Description of the current version of the approach*

Figure 12.1 presents our tool-based approach for a retrospective analysis in seven steps. The agent who applies it cannot be the OR manager since the latter cannot stop working. Steps 2–7 must be carried out one to two days after the observation day (step 1) in order to be able to provide immediate feedback to the OR manager and the operating suite agents (step 7).

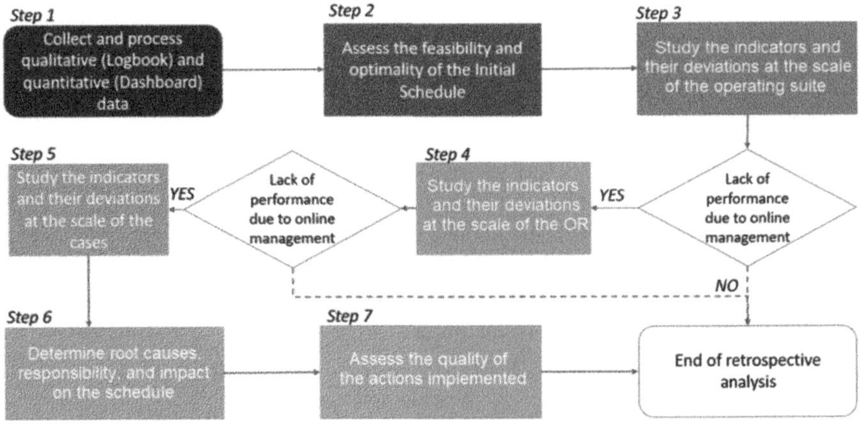

Figure 12.1. *Flowchart presenting the different stages of our retrospective analysis approach. For a color version of this figure, see www.iste.co.uk/chaabane/healthcare.zip*

12.3.3.1. *Step 1 – collect and process qualitative and quantitative data*

The objective of this step is to collect and process the qualitative and quantitative data related to the operating day we wish to analyze. To this end, it is necessary to update the Logbook (tool 1) throughout the day and run the Dashboard (tool 2) once the schedule execution is over.

12.3.3.2. *Step 2 – assess the feasibility and optimality of the initial schedule*

The inconsistencies of the IS and lack of respect for the basic scheduling rules can cause deviations and prevent the target values of the performance indicators from being achieved. We have defined a list of assumptions to be respected in order to avoid inconsistencies and reduce the potential of suboptimal scheduling. These assumptions must be followed in order to distinguish between deviations from scheduling and from online management. We take it for granted that the scheduling is done so that the IS is optimal.

Table 12.4 shows the two types of assumptions to be respected throughout scheduling: Consistency Hypothesis (CH) and Performance Hypothesis (PH). These are based on the specific local solutions of the operating suite at the CHN and may change from one operating suite to another. The verification of these hypotheses can be integrated into the operating suite management in the form of indicators, in order to facilitate detection.

Hypothesis	Drafting assistance
CH#1	The first case begins at least 15 minutes after the opening of the AOT so that the staff have time to "open" the OR.
CH#2	There is time dedicated for OR clean-up after each intervention.
PH#1	There is no scheduled intervention outside of AOT hours.
PH#2	There is no scheduled time between two cases.

Table 12.4. *Hypothetical assumptions to be respected throughout scheduling*

12.3.3.3. *Step 3 – study the indicators and their deviations at the scale of the operating suite*

During steps 3–5, the indicators and their deviations are studied at three respective scales, starting from the operating suite up to the case itself. In step 3, we thus limit ourselves to the scope of the operating suite and determine whether it is relevant to deepen our analysis through a study of the ORs. First, at the scale of the operating suite, we calculate indicators for IS and PS as well as any deviations between the two schedules. Next, we study whether they reach the targets as set out by the ANAP and interpret the results obtained. The analysis process is continued if the PS indicators do not reach their target and/or if the deviations are potentially due to online management.

12.3.3.4. *Step 4 – study the indicators and their deviations at the scale of the operating room*

If the indicators and the deviations aggregated at the block level from step 3 have identified a lack of performance then these are studied in step 4, room by room. In this case, there is at least one indicator per room that does not meet its target. This step is similar to step 3 except that the values are calculated at the OR level. The process is continued if the deviations are potentially attributable to the OR manager.

12.3.3.5. *Step 5 – study the indicators and their deviations at the scale of the cases*

Step 5 is applied to each OR for which there is at least one indicator that does not reach its target or for which the deviations potentially depend on the OR manager in place. In this chapter, for each intervention in each room concerned, we only study the following durations: late start, early end, restricted overtime, waiting for cleaning and waiting for patient. We note the initial durations used to calculate our base indicators from Table 12.2. For each of the times identified, we note its ID, its nature, its milestones and its characteristic duration. If possible, indicate the function normally responsible for preventing the deviation from occurring, in order to be able to analyze – if necessary – whether the tools provided are suitable or whether the IS is in fact achievable.

12.3.3.6. *Step 6 – determine the root causes, the responsibility and the impact on the schedule*

To begin with, we combine the information from the Dashboard and the Logbook to identify the root causes and the function to which the deviations and/or malfunctions are attributed. Next, we characterize their impact on the PS in the form of unavoidable/avoidable advances or delays. For example, if the IS has the first intervention at 8 a.m. then a preparation delay will be inevitable. On the other hand, patient entry delays due to the fact that nurses are scheduled for a break are avoidable.

12.3.3.7. *Step 7 – assess the quality of the actions implemented*

In this step, we assess how the OR manager dealt with the deviations; we note the action carried out as well as its evaluation. We only study those that are attributable to it or potentially attributable to it. The analysis takes place in three stages: (1) check that the OR manager has detected the deviations and identify the actions they took in order to take charge of them; (2) compare these actions to the root causes identified; and (3) assess the quality of the person responsible, depending on the severity of the impact of the deviation on the OR schedule. To this end, we can apply the temporal deviation or milestones as well as the indicators described in Table 12.2. All of the information concerning the actions and decisions of the OR manager is in the Logbook. The rest can be found in both tools.

EXAMPLE.– Here is an example summary of steps 5–7 for a disruption: (ID: 2, nature: clean-up delay, milestones: 11:25 a.m. – 11:35 a.m., duration: 10 min, root cause: that the ORAs are on a break, responsibility is: attributable to online management, impacts are: avoidable delays, action: go and inform the ORAs that the patient has left the room, assessment: relevant action but the delay could have been avoided if the OR manager had warned the ORAs beforehand). ORA is the acronym for the OR Assistant, who is in charge of cleaning up the ORs.

Once the data collection, processing and analysis are complete, the agent in charge of carrying out the approach can present these results to the OR manager and the operating suite agents. The objective is multiple: make staff aware of good practices, objectify the feelings of employees, remove performance barriers, etc.

12.4. Applied example of our tool-based approach at the *Centre Hospitalier de Narbonne*

12.4.1. *Step 1 – collect and process the data*

In the context of this example, we are studying the schedule execution of a 6-OR operating suite over the course of one day. We focus our observations on the hours of the OR manager's shift, that is, from 8:00 a.m. to 3:30 p.m. We have populated the Logbook as shown in Table 12.3. Table 12.5 describes the two disruptions that we use in this example. We also ran the Dashboard in order to be able to calculate all of our indicators and their deviations.

	Disruption 1	**Disruption 2**	**No.**
ID	3	4	1
Detection time	10:37 a.m.	11:53 a.m.	2
Description	Patient #2 in OR#2 is waiting for their locoregional anesthesia (LRA) to be performed	Case #2 in OR#2 has not yet started	3
Impact on the schedule	Risk of delay if the LRA is not done on time	Risk of delaying the start of case #2	4
Root causes	The anesthesiologist is not available	The clean-up of the previous case has not started	5
Time	Three actions at (1) 10:37 a.m. (2) 10:43 a.m. and (3) 11:43 a.m.	No action	6
Description	(1) Ask the nurses of the recovery room where the anesthesiologist is, (2, 3) Check if the patient has received their LRA	No action	7
Outcome	(1) The anesthesiologist is expected to arrive soon, (2) No, (3) Yes	No action	8

Table 12.5. *Example of Logbook entries for disruptions (lines 1–5) and actions taken to remedy them (lines 6–8)*

12.4.2. *Step 2 – evaluate the feasibility and optimality of the initial schedule*

We checked the feasibility and optimality assumptions for the IS of each room. IH#1 is not respected: all of the first cases are scheduled at the opening time of the session. Therefore, there will necessarily be a late start in the PS. The other assumptions are partially respected: 4 interventions out of 31 do not have any clean-up assigned, 2 ORs have a restricted overtime of 5 min and 24 min, respectively, and 5 cases are followed by an unoccupied shift time.

12.4.3. *Steps 3 and 4 – study the indicators and their deviations for the operating suite and the operating rooms*

A study of the operating suite indicators reveals that not all of them reached their performance targets (step 3). In order to respect the size constraints, we will continue the analysis on OR#2 only, an orthopedic OR whose performance indicators do not all reach their target, and for which only the IH#1 hypothesis was not respected. We calculated the deviations of base indicators and duration indicators, shown in Table 12.6.

Indicators	Target	IS	PS	Deviation
Utilization rate (UR)	85%	91%	88%	–3%
Late start rate (LSR)	<5%	0%	2%	**+2%**
Early stop rate (ESR)	<5%	**9%**	0%	–9%
Restricted overtime rate (ROR)	<5%	0%	5%	**+5%**
Time between cases rate (BCR)	<5%	0%	**10%**	**+10%**
Surgery Duration (SD)	/	7h20	8h	+40min (+7% AOT)
Clean-up duration (CUD)	/	1h31	2h	+29min (+5% AOT)
Case duration (CD)	/	8h51	10h	+69min (+12% AOT)

Table 12.6. *Indicators and their deviations. The ratios are in bold if they do not reach their targets (IS and PS) or if there is a deterioration from the IS to the PS (deviation)*

Here, we briefly comment on the results. From Table 12.6, we went from 9% idle time at the end of a shift to 5% overtime. In other words: the IS was set to finish early while the PS ended late. A question then arises: Would it have been possible to finish the cases before the end of the AOT despite the IS? We want to know whether it was possible to have a Restricted Overtime Rate of 0%. For that, we study unoccupied shift times. The 2% Late Start Rate is not compressible. The

Time Between Case Rate achieved reached 10% (a deviation of + 10%) and exceeded the target by at least 5%. This deviation could potentially absorb the 5% Restricted Overtime Rate. Therefore, the goal of this analysis is to identify what caused at least 5% deviation in the Time Between Case Rate and determine whether or not it could have been avoided.

12.4.4. *Step 5 – study the indicators and their deviations at the level of the interventions*

This section summarizes step 5 of our approach. To simplify the study, we neither note the deviations after the end of the OR manager's shift nor do we take into account the restricted overtime. We identify four deviations at the scale of the case: one late start (ID#1, 13 min, 8:00 a.m. – 8:13 a.m.), one wait for cleaning (ID#2, 18 min, 11:36 a.m. – 11:54 a.m.) and two patient expectations (ID#3, 10 min, 12:15 a.m. –12:25 a.m.; ID#4, 6 min, 1:20 p.m. – 1:26 p.m.).

12.4.5. *Step 6 – determine root causes, impact on the performed schedule and responsibility for deviations*

With the data contained in our tools and in the schedule, we can identify: (i) the root causes, (ii) the responsibility for each deviation and (iii) the deviation impact on the PS. We present the results of step 6 in Table 12.7 below.

ID	Root cause	Responsibility	Impact on the performed schedule
1	IH #1 not respected and therefore the IS is not achievable	Scheduling	**Inevitable delay.** Risk of overestimating the Allocated OR Time in the initial schedule
2	The order of the clean-ups is not optimal	Online Management	**Potentially avoidable delay** with another order to clean the rooms (OR#2 then OR#5) or a division of the ORA team
3	Unknown	Unknown for the moment	**Potentially avoidable delay** of 10 min if the deviation had been noticed.
4	Deviation inherent to the schedule execution	None	**Inevitable delay** inherent to the schedule execution

Table 12.7. *Summary of step 6*

12.4.6. *Step 7 – evaluate the quality of the actions implemented*

This section presents the analysis of the intersection of information between deviations attributable, or potentially attributable, to online management and information on disruptions described in the Logbook. The OR manager has detected deviation #2 (clean-up delay) but it was too late for any action to be taken. If they had detected the deviation in time, they could have, for example, maintained the cleaning order for the ORs and asked the ORA to form two teams. As a result, the 18-minute delay could have been avoided. Deviation #3 was not detected by the OR manager. If they had detected it, they could have informed the nurses that it was possible to get the next patient into the OR and the delay would therefore have potentially been avoided. No action was taken for either of these deviations.

12.4.7. *Summation*

The objective of this analysis was to determine the root causes of at least 5% of the Time Between Case Rate and determine whether it was in fact compressible. The value of the Between Intervention Rate achieved is 10%. It was caused by five deviations occurring during the shift, three of which occurred during the OR manager's shift (6% of the Inter-intervention Rate): ID#2 was avoidable (3%), ID#3 was potentially avoidable (2%) and ID#4 was not preventable (1%). As shown in the previous steps, ID#2 was detected too late to make a change and ID#3 was not detected at all. We could have reduced the Time Between Intervention Rate by a maximum of 5% and avoided any Restricted Overtime through different management (e.g. by improving the process of detecting deviations in real time). However, as some deviations were only potentially avoidable, we cannot confirm this. We also showed that the IS was not optimal.

12.5. Conclusion and perspectives

Random disruptions and schedule deviations are inherent in activity that takes place in the operating suite, in which the human factor is dominant. As part of this study, we have gradually built a retrospective tool-based approach allowing us to: (1) analyze the deviations between the IS and the PS, and (2) assess the way in which the online management handled them. The example presented highlights the potential added value of this approach. Our work has shown that improvements can be made in both the construction and execution of the schedule. Improvements could include more frequent patient pathway checks and a decision support system for the OR manager. The possible consequences of this study are multiple: extend the scope of the study to the entire operating suite, add indicators (turnover, delay in milestones, etc.) and semi-automate the process of collecting, processing and analyzing data.

12.6. References

ANAP (2016a). Bloc opératoire – établir une planification adaptée [Online]. Available at: http://bloc-operatoire.anap.fr/publication/1258-etablir-une-planification-adaptee.

ANAP (2016b). Bloc opératoire – liste des indicateurs fréquemment suivis dans les blocs [Online]. Available at: http://bloc-operatoire.anap.fr/publication/1297.

Aniba, S. and Jebali, A. (2011). Approches stochastiques pour la planification des interventions au bloc opératoire. *CIGI*, 8.

Chaabane, S., Meskens, N., Guinet, A., Laurent, M. (2007). Comparaison des performances des politiques de programmation opératoire. *Logistique & Management*, 15(1), 17–26.

Gentil, S. (2013). Les "agencements organisationnels" des situations perturbées : la coordination d'un bloc opératoire à la pointe de la rationalisation industrielle. *Communiquer. Revue de communication sociale et publique*, 65–80.

Hammami, S., Ladet, P., Atidel, B.H.A., Ruiz, A. (2007). Une programmation opératoire robuste. *Logistique & Management*, 15(1), 95–111.

Koppka, L., Wiesche, L., Schacht, M., Werners, B. (2018). Optimal distribution of operating hours over operating rooms using probabilities. *European Journal of Operational Research*, 267(3), 1156–1171.

Macario, A. (2006). Are your hospital operating rooms "efficient"? A scoring system with eight performance indicators. *Anesthesiology*, 105(2), 237–240.

Macario, A., Vitez, T.S., Dunn, B., McDonald, T., Brown, B. (1997). Hospital costs and severity of illness in three types of elective surgery. *Anesthesiology*, 86(1), 92–100.

Pauchard, E. (2010). 5 Pourquoi et QQOQCP – deux outils indispensables [Online]. Available at: http://www.eponine-pauchard.com/2010/06/5-pourquoi-et-qqoqcp/.

Samudra, M., Van Riet, C., Demeulemeester, E., Cardoen, B., Vansteenkiste, N., Rademakers, F.E. (2016). Scheduling operating rooms: Achievements, challenges and pitfalls. *Journal of Scheduling*, 19(5), 493–525.

Tancrez, J.-S., Roland, B., Cordier, J.-P., Riane, F. (2011). Étude de la perturbation par les urgences du planning opératoire. *Logistique & Management*, 19(2), 43–52.

13

Planning Patient Journeys in Outpatient Hospitals to Support the Ambulatory Shift

13.1. Introduction

Patient care in hospitals has evolved rapidly and has sometimes been at odds with hospital organizations. As Burnel (2017) noted, despite the reform of T2A (Activity-Based Costing or ABC), institutions "have not thoroughly revised their processes and organizations, contenting themselves with adjustment measures on variable costs". The recent law grouping hospitals under a common medical project is the last hurdle towards the standardization of hospital structures, which is *a priori* at odds with the societal and financial changes that stimulate the hospital to provide shorter, less expensive and more condensed care, in closer connection with the city. The initiatives for the reduction of the Average Length of Stay (ALOS), Enhanced Recovery After Surgery (ERAS), Day 0/Day 1 units, ambulatory shift and outpatient clinics are the continuous elements of this evolution. The difficulty is that the public hospital must develop these short-stay structures, while maintaining a high level of technicality, so as to treat the most serious and urgent cases, mixing a dense scheduled flow with a significant unscheduled flow.

A profound organizational transformation is therefore necessary, in which flow monitoring must play an important role: patient flows are varied, and suitable methodologies must be considered. For example, if the outpatient flow can be planned better, it must also be monitored. This implies transposing industrial planning and monitoring procedures to specific hospital features, in order to offer healthcare providers simple and effective methods to achieve this. We are particularly interested in the developments of outpatient medicine, through dedicated clinics, and we have developed a macro-planning routine for a Sales and Operation

Chapter written by Virginie FORTINEAU and Lucie ROUSSEL.

Plan (S&Op), in order to help institutions correctly estimate their resources and plan patient journeys.

After addressing the issue of patient flows and existing flow management methods, we will show the importance of these approaches, and the current lack of proposals for tactical patient flow planning in the literature. We contribute to this with a method of macro-planning for groups of pathways, adapted to three real-world cases, and finally, we discuss the limits and perspectives of this methodology for outpatient medical structures.

13.2. Background and state-of-the-art methods

13.2.1. *Planning patient journeys at the hospital*

The public hospital faces organizational challenges in managing its patient flows. At a hospital site, different kinds of patient flows coexist, from outpatient consultations, to the management of major emergencies (shock, multiple traumas, etc.). From an organizational point of view, this leads to a contradictory injunction, formulated, on the one hand, by the requirement of efficiency and low costs with regard to the flows open to the city and, on the other hand, by the need for highly technical and responsive staff to manage vital emergencies, perform "primary" surgery and innovate. The diagram below shows the different types of hospital flows, from the most repeatable (i.e. plannable) to the least predictable (i.e. in need of monitoring). Therefore, each category of patient flow must make use of planning and monitoring methods that have been adapted differently.

However, hospitals are not used to the planning and monitoring methods. Hospitals more readily use the nebulous term "programming", a one-size-fits-all term that often covers a little of both concepts, but only partially: planning often comes down to making an appointment on an *ad hoc* basis, and guiding this scheduling inevitably results in an inexorable series of untimely cancellations, and rarely the multidisciplinary and enlightened decision-making that is sought after. One of the factors for this deficiency is methodological, as the hospital rarely has the necessary prerequisites for planning and monitoring flows. In addition to the lack of skills in flow management within hospital profiles (all units combined), we note that:

– to direct is to act, and we can only act on what we see. The prerequisite for monitoring flows is therefore to view the status of the system in real time, which is not the case in all hospitals;

– planning is forecasting: the establishment of forecasts and standardized technical data is therefore essential. While it is possible to obtain activity forecasts, working off estimated lengths of stay and the standard patient journeys, it remains a challenge for an environment wherein it is common to hear that "each patient is different".

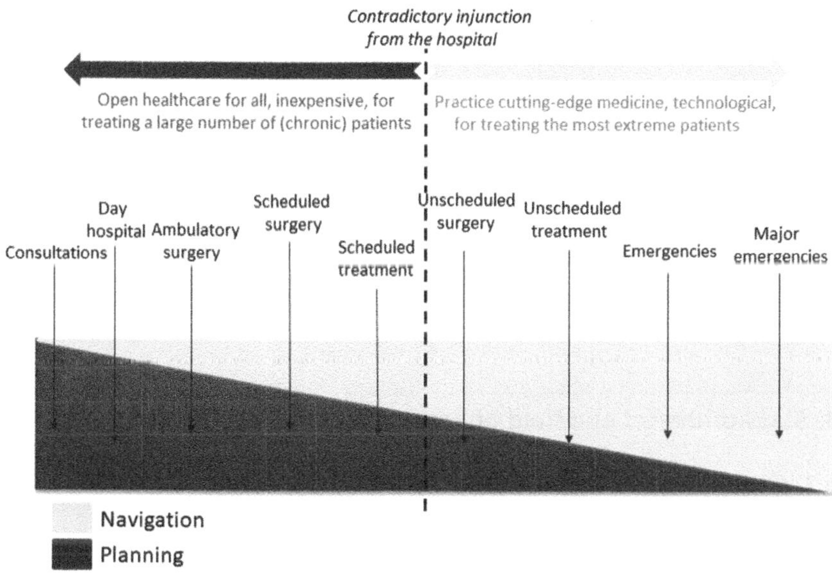

Figure 13.1. *Breakdown for types of patient flows. For a color version of this figure, see www.iste.co.uk/chaabane/healthcare.zip*

Finally, the ultimate limiting factor is that it is not enough to apply robust industry methodologies as a solution to the hospital planning problem, as patient flow is by its very nature different to a manufacturing flow (as demonstrated by Fortineau *et al.* (2017)), which renders industry tools inapplicable as they follow a specific methodology and therefore need rethinking.

13.2.2. *4.0 transforming the operational management of hospital flows*

On the issue of flow monitoring and direction, things are changing with the arrival of 4.0 technologies. From the point of view of organization flows, the early 4.0 technologies, such as RFID, have brought significant advances in the real-time knowledge of systems, as well as other revolutionary amendments for flow management in the hospital. Note, in particular, the introduction of RFID wristbands for patients, very advanced in the United States, which allows an instant update of the patient location/status, or a real-time follow-up of the patient's journey through the operating rooms. Such technologies are also used on equipment (stretchers and stretcher chairs, biomedical equipment, etc.) to facilitate flow management and control logistical flows (RFID KANBAN, RFID-Enabled Cabinets, oxygen cylinder tracing, etc.). Despite all these advances in operational flow monitoring, the question of planning remains little explored. This is the objective of this work.

13.2.3. *Research problem*

The research problem is therefore to develop a planning methodology for repeatable patient flows, so as to avoid scenarios of managing "noise", and instead improve the hospital organizations. This method must be robust, adapted to the specificity of patient flows, and suitable for use by healthcare personnel. As an example of a plannable patient flow, we have chosen outpatient medicine, which is currently growing.

13.3. State-of-the-art and field of application

13.3.1. *Field of application: patient flows in outpatient hospitals*

Outpatient care provides standardized care and is governed at the national level by regulations, which stipulate the minimal content of hospitalizations that may generate – within the framework of costings based on the activities (ABCs or T2As in French) – a flat rate, generally between 400 € and 700 € per outpatient. If the regulations are not respected (e.g. if one of the radiological examinations is missing), the outpatient care will be paid on a fee-for-service basis, which represents a financial loss. This economic constraint increases the stakes *vis-à-vis* taking care of the patient at all steps of their ambulatory care: indeed, a postponement of an examination due to disorganization will have – in addition to impacts on the quality of care – pecuniary consequences, which can be dramatic in the long run.

To properly support these outpatient facilities, hospitals are creating dedicated, multidisciplinary ambulatory medical structures that take place on reproducible typical days. There are two distinct categories of flows among all of these pathways:

– So-called "long" courses, such as chemotherapy cures, where the patient is "confined" to their seat. They stay in their seat or in their outpatient room for most of the day. This requires continuous monitoring, and therefore, several patients can be taken care of by the same staff at the same time (e.g. a nurse looks after a given number of chemotherapy chairs).

– So-called "short" courses, because the patient does not spend much time in an outpatient chair they will undergo a series of tests, examinations and interviews, some of which take place outside the ambulatory facility. For example, a diagnostic pathway will involve assessments taken from the outpatient facility, such as a medical interview with the day hospital doctor on duty, but it may also require a scan to be carried out by a neighboring radiology department. These pathways require a lot of programming, and involve a variety of health professionals, part of whom may be external to the hospital (e.g. physiotherapist and orthoptists).

Both of these types of pathways need to be planned; however, we are especially interested in the latter, as they are more complex from a flow management point of view.

With regard to the hospital organization, the development of shared reception structures for outpatient medicine constitutes a profound change. These new structures, the size of which is only growing in order to comply with efficiency requirements, imply a complexification of the patient flow, and thus require real engineering tools. However, the organizational challenge of, for example, the daily coordination of two to three outpatients in a conventional service, is not the same as, for example, managing a multidisciplinary outpatient clinic that processes 40 patients per day. It is out of the question, on this scale, to schedule all patients at 8 a.m., or to request radiological examinations one by one, without creating daily difficulties for the staff involved. In addition, the outpatient must leave by the evening of that same day, with all of their examinations carried out, and a medical summary. As such, an outpatient structure that is not organized will become a deficit factory for the hospital, and will be a source of suffering for the staff.

13.3.2. *Little tactical planning for the state of the art*

To establish the state-of-the-art framework analysis, we have chosen to rely on industrial classifications of flow management methods. These methods, grouped under the terminology OMPs (Operations Management Practices), can be classified according to four types:

1) Methods for the planning/scheduling of Manufacturing Resources Planning (MRP2).

2) Pull-flow management methods based on Lean Manufacturing.

3) The theory of constraints, and the methods for navigating by constraints, in general.

4) Decision-making, optimization and/or simulation methods, such as Petri networks, and algorithms.

We also classified contributions according to their level of application: from operational to strategic. Finally, the last classification criterion is whether they are outpatient structures with long-term pathways (e.g. chemotherapy, in gray) or mixed structures, including short-term pathways.

	Planning/ Scheduling	Pull-flow (Lean)/TOC	Simulation/ Decision-making	
Strategic	Bonvin *et al.* 2009		Vahdat *et al.* 2019	13%
Tactical	Gunawan and Lau 2013		Villamizar *et al.* 2011	20%
			Tohidi *et al.* 2019	
			Aeenparast *et al.* 2013	
Operational		Sadki 2012	Santibáñez *et al.* 2009	60%
		Compondu *et al.* 2018	Ahmed 2011	
		Klasen *et al.* 2014	Gupta 2011	
		Lamé *et al.* 2016	Cayirli *et al.* 2006	
			Green 2007	
	13%	27%	60%	

Figure 13.2. *Classification of planning inputs for outpatient medicine. For a color version of this figure, see www.iste.co.uk/chaabane/healthcare.zip*

The vast majority of publications focus on the operations level, offering detailed organization optimizations through simulations or *ad hoc* mathematical optimization models. Even when the results resemble tactical planning decisions, they are obtained through the generalization of simulated operations scenarios (Aeenparast *et al.* 2013; Tohidi *et al.* 2019). These contributions can be criticized for their very mathematical approach to hospital management, not contributing to the development of tools applicable to beginners (the caregivers themselves). In addition, a large part of these contributions are not concerned with the organization of healthcare, but with arranging an appointment and the time it takes to achieve it (Cayirli *et al.* 2006; Green *et al.* 2007; Gupta 2012).

Since the 2010s, Lean approaches have complemented mathematical models, particularly in the case of chemotherapy hospitals. In 2016, chemotherapy still represented 80% of daycare pathways (Lamé *et al.* 2016). They require the production of treatment bags by the hospital pharmacy, and therefore, there needs to be synchronization between these two flows, which involves "Lean" organizational projects, such as that of the Antoine-Béclère hospital (Klasen *et al.* 2014), or that covered in the study by Lamé *et al.* (2016). Chemotherapy day hospitals present a problem for flow management that is different from ours. It is less complicated to plan than short-term pathways, however, it also comes with its own set of challenges, in particular, the strict reoccurrence of treatments. For these reasons, the solutions for chemotherapy day hospitals, if they serve as a source of inspiration, cannot be transposed directly to ambulatory medicine in the broader sense.

It is not surprising that Lean implementation approaches in day hospitals focus on the operational level, because Lean is a method for managing operational flows. However, it is astonishing to note the bibliographical vacuum on the tactical planning of this type of structure. Only the study by Gunawan and Lau (2013) proposes the implementation of a Master Production Schedule (MPS), but on a larger scale than the day hospital. Then, there are the other contributions to planning that focus on very strategic levels, such as that of the Swiss cantons by Bonvin *et al.* (2009), which applied macro-planning to the field of psychiatry.

13.3.3. *Choosing a planning and workflow management method*

It seems important to us to propose tactical planning approaches for outpatient medicine, because otherwise, the operational mathematical models are forced to optimize not the natural hazards of the system, but a lot of the "noise" instead: in short, all of the dysfunctions generated by the absence of tactical anticipation (i.e. the correct sizing), thus complicating the problem. All the more so since patient flows in outpatient medicine are different from other patient flows in hospitals, as shown in Figure 13.1: they are predictable, standardizable and plannable. We know the patient's planned treatments (prescription) in advance, which are generally repeatable from one patient to another for the same pathology, and we can predict the queues by pathway type.

Another characteristic of the flow in ambulatory medicine that requires planning is that the flow must be anticipated:

– for chronic patients, who are still active, and therefore need to plan ahead for time off to visit the day hospital;

– for professionals, since it often calls on "external" staff and non-dedicated internal resources, which must therefore be allocated in advance.

For all of these reasons, we were interested in the MRP2 methodology, which is an approach that was conceived in the 1970s and implemented in Enterprise Resource Planning (ERP) type information systems that are widely used in the industry. It offers continuous progression from a macro-planning, called a Sales and Operations Plan (S&Op), to the detailed management of the workshop applied throughout the life cycle of Manufacturing Orders (MOs) and Purchase Orders (POs) (Baglin *et al.* 2015). Initially, we explored the principle of the S&Op and the Master Production Schedule (MPS), which allows for tactical planning, an essential articulation allowing for strategies and organizational HR models predetermined upstream to be transformed into efficient support at the operational level. This level, as expressed previously, faces a lack of scientific literature at present.

13.4. Contribution

13.4.1. *Macro-planning for groups of pathways: an S&Op for ambulatory medicine*

We have transposed the principle of S&Op to MRP2 methodology for use in day hospital medicine. The proposed approach thus consists, analogously to the S&Op, a macro-planning (macro-planning of pathways for groups of pathways) based on patient journey groups. The input data required for the macro-planning of pathway groups is:

– patient journeys (see Figure 13.3), which correspond to the articles, routines and bill-of-materials of MPR2;

– activity forecasts;

– the constitution of groups of pathways;

– all of the resources (human, material, etc.) and their capacities.

The first step in the implementation of the macro-planning for groups of pathways is the quantified stream mapping of the patient pathway, discussed in Fortineau *et al.* (2017). This is a major step in the organization process, as it encourages the formalization and standardization of healthcare, a *sine qua non* for the efficient organization of an outpatient clinic.

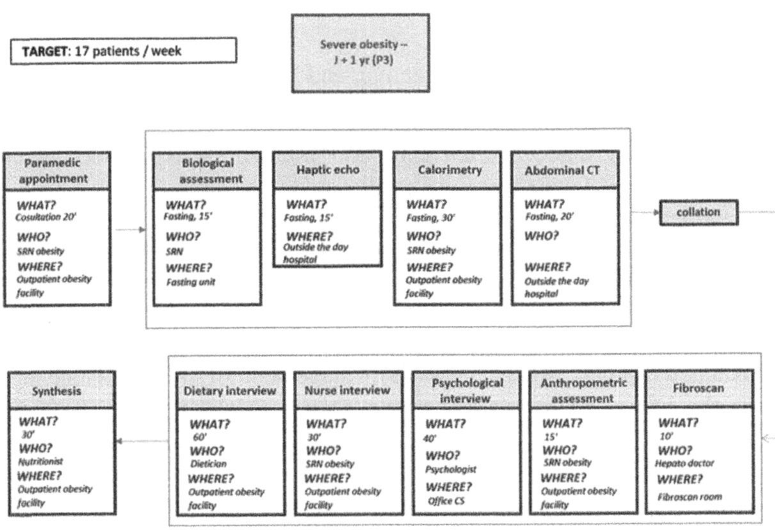

Figure 13.3. *A quantified stream mapping of patient pathway, essential technical data for the macro-planning for groups of pathways. For a color version of this figure, see www.iste.co.uk/chaabane/healthcare.zip*

The activity targets for each pathway, grouped together in order to simplify the planning approach, can then be compared to actual resource capacities, leading to organizational changes. Indeed, the objective of pathway modeling is to make it possible to calculate the overall loads on each type of resource, in order to compare them with the resources available. This load/capacity ratio is expressed in Figure 13.4. The number of patients expected for each family of pathways is reported on each line. Knowing the detailed quantified patient pathways makes it possible to calculate the occupancy time of each resource. We are particularly interested in bottleneck resources, which can be human, or any other type, such as imagery equipment. This first comparison also makes it possible to determine the days when it is possible to complete the pathway (the criterion is that all of the necessary resources must be present on that day). As the calculation is dynamic, it is possible to "play" with the organizations (resources or distribution of patients), in order to achieve a load smoothing, of a standard week of the ambulatory unit. Reasoning through groups of pathways makes it possible to simplify the sizing process, which at this level is multidisciplinary, and therefore aims to get the various ambulatory specialties involved in the outpatient structure to work together.

		Monday		Tuesday		Wednesday		Thursday		Friday		Realised	TARGET
	Group 1: obesity	9	OK	9	OK	9	OK	9	OK	9	OK	45	51
	Group 2: chemotherapy	11	OK	11	OK	11	OK	11	OK	11	OK	55	55
	Group 3: long-term	5	OK	5	OK	6	OK	10	OK	10	OK	36	36
Geriatrics	Recollection and assessment		IMP	1	OK		IMP		IMP	5	OK	6	6
	Nutrition		IMP	0	OK		IMP		IMP	0	OK	0	1
	Decline		IMP	2	OK		IMP		IMP		IMP	2	2
	Group 5: short-term	15	OK	15	OK	11	OK	10	OK	9	OK	60	60
	Rheumatology		IMP		IMP		IMP		IMP	2	OK	2	2
Group 6: diabetes	Assessment of complications	4	OK		IMP	0	OK		IMP		IMP	4	4
	Etiological diagnostic assessment	2	OK		IMP	3	OK		IMP		IMP	5	3
	Diabetic foot		IMP		IMP	3	OK		IMP		IMP	3	3
	Insulin pump, holter, diabetic	P diabe	IMP		IMP		IMP		IMP		IMP	0	1
	Group 7: neurology		IMP	4	OK		IMP		IMP		IMP	4	4
	Group 8: cardiology		IMP		IMP		IMP		IMP		IMP	0	7
		46										222	235

	Monday		Tuesday		Wednesday		Thursday		Friday	
Social worker	0.00	0%	0.28	4%	0.00	0%	0.00	0%	1.39	19%
Generalist SRN	16.11	72%	17.70	74%	14.77	70%	17.14	70%	18.87	77%
Obesity SRN	12.37	82%	12.37	82%	12.37	82%	12.37	82%	12.37	82%
Chemotherapy SRN	11.92	79%	11.92	79%	11.92	79%	11.92	79%	11.92	79%
Dressings SRN	0.00	ABS	0.00	0%	2.00	37%	0.00	0%	0.00	0%
Diabetes SRN	1.00	27%	0.00	ABS	1.50	40%	0.00	ABS	0.00	ABS
Neurologist	0.00	ABS	4.42	110%	0.00	ABS	0.00	ABS	0.00	ABS
Psychologist	5.63	70%	6.13	77%	5.63	70%	5.63	70%	5.63	70%

Figure 13.4. *Impact of the macro-planning for groups of pathways on resources (occupancy rate). For a color version of this figure, see www.iste.co.uk/chaabane/healthcare.zip*

It is thus imperative to make this a recurring approach (every six months, for example) and multidisciplinary, making it possible to reach a consensus between the different medical specialties, and provide credibility to the coordination team of the outpatient structure which will be responsible for the operational implementation of this macro-planning.

13.4.2. *Feedback*

We formulated and developed this approach based on three very different applied case studies. The first was the pooling of all the day facilities of a hospital into a common unit, bringing together seven medical specialties, based around 25 standard patient pathways, with an activity target of 40 patients per day. For this applied case study, the size of the ambulatory structure to be built required objectified and quantified modeling, which made it difficult to "build by hand". The main contributions of this approach to the teams were to facilitate the definition of the architectural program by objectifying the use of the premises and the sizing of the human resources to be considered, and also to foster team spirit within the ambulatory structure, which was dedicated to bringing together pathways that previously existed in isolation within each medical service. The professionals understood that there needed to be a formal organization, which was not the result of their past organizations (smoothing over the week, in particular), leading to organizational transformations.

The second case was the programming of the day hospital and the weekly hospital of a neuropediatric department that was in difficulty at the time (many programming delays). The approach made it possible to understand that a large part of the pathways were not feasible because they involved too many resources that were not available at the same time, which led to the creation of simpler sub-routes, and to the modification of the shift days of two neuropsychologists. It also enabled a factual discussion on pre-dedicated imaging appointments (for example, MRI scans were reserved every Monday from 10am to 12 am), a fundamental input in the organization of outpatient day hospitals.

The last case study was the creation of a programming cell typical to neurology day hospitals, which were then divided into three different departments. The process, led by the State Registered Nurse (SRN) coordinator, helped to structure the organizations, especially the roles of agents in the new programming unit, providing them with planning procedures and tools. The results have been an increase in monthly schedules, reduced processing times and overall increase in activities.

13.5. Discussion and perspectives

13.5.1. *Repeatability and accessibility of the macro-planning approach*

The macro-planning approach is accessible to caregivers after a short adjustment period, which allows them to take ownership. In all three case studies, the healthcare teams have gained their independence using the tool. The test on three different structures showed the significant repeatability of this macro-planning step. The only limitation found is that of the third structure studied, which had the particularity of ambulatory shifts over two days, without *a priori* distribution of activities between these two days. Since the proposed modeling did not cover this case study, a standard distribution was applied in order to reduce the problem to that of two consecutive ambulatory shifts. The other difficulty for the caregivers is the grouping of pathways, which they tend to do from a pathological point of view, when it is important to group the treatments in terms of the similarities in the stages and allocation of resources, even though the pathologies are very different.

13.5.2. *Beyond the macro-planning for groups of pathways: towards integrated planning*

The resulting forecast of the macro-planning for groups of pathways must then be implemented at the operational level. If the macro-planning for groups of pathways is a multidisciplinary step, the rest of the process is the responsibility of the coordination team of the outpatient structure. Based on the macro-planning for groups of pathways, it is necessary to develop day-to-day schedules, taking into account specific constraints: vacations, scheduled maintenance and so on, in short, translating the macro-planning for groups of pathways into a Master Production Schedule (MPS) that we call "planning detailed pathway" (see Figure 13.5). Each typical outpatient day is then broken down, activity by activity. Depending on the size of the structure and the type of flow, this can be done by hand, using charts, or by using a scheduling engine, should the problem be too complex. The scheduling results give a detailed schedule for a typical day, with an arrival time and the pathway of examinations for each treatment. Then, the coordinating SRNs can position, according to the prescriptions of the doctors, the patients into these pre-established standard slots (the POs). This saves them from having to make plans for patients one by one, which often leads to poor results, because the interactions between patient pathways (scheduling problem) have not been taken into account.

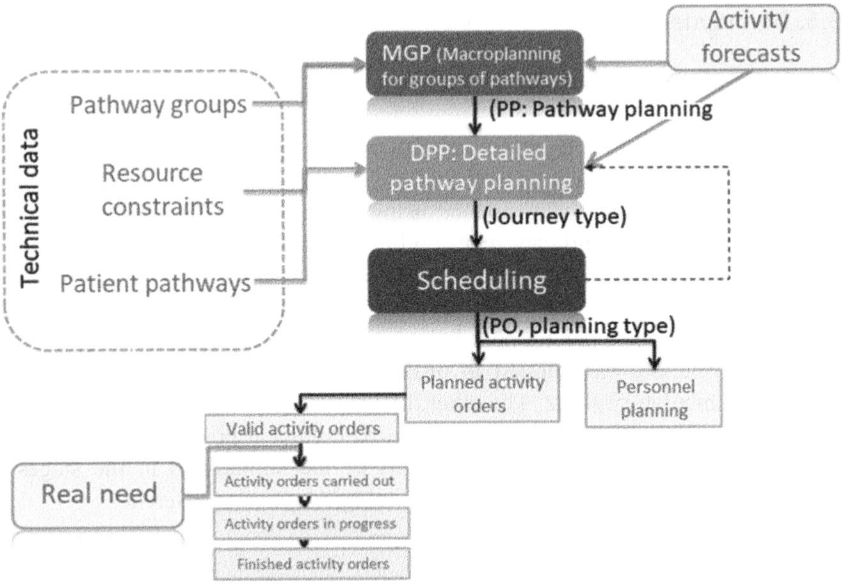

Figure 13.5. *Process and adaptation of integrated planning (MRP2) for ambulatory patient journeys. For a color version of this figure, see www.iste.co.uk/chaabane/healthcare.zip*

13.6. Conclusion

To meet the challenges of shifting to ambulatory care, the public hospital must change the organizational paradigm of its day hospitals and integrate the importance of planning into flow management. The construction of dedicated ambulatory platforms is an element of this transformation, which must be accompanied by effective organizational methods, and in particular, tactical planning. With the macro-planning for groups of pathways (a transposition of the S&Op method), outpatient facilities have a simple, understandable and repeatable tool that allows them to properly estimate their resources and the reception of patients. This tool must, in the future, be accompanied by detailed planning methods and coordinate with the necessary operational management of flows.

13.7. References

Aeenparast, A., Tabibi, S.J., Shahanaghi, K., Aryanejhad, M.B. (2013). Reducing outpatient waiting time: A simulation modeling approach. *Iranian Red Crescent Medical Journal*, 15(9), 865.

Ahmed, Z., ElMekkawy, T.Y., Bates, S. (2011). Developing an efficient scheduling template of a chemotherapy treatment unit: A case study. *The Australasian Medical Journal*, 4(10), 575.

Baglin, G., Lamouri, S., Thomas, A. (2015). *Maîtriser les logiciels ERP*. Editions Economica, Paris, France.

Bonvin, E., Basterrechea, L., Guex, P. (2009). Psychiatrie sous double contrainte, enjeux de la planification en santé mentale. *Revue médicale suisse*, 5, 217.

Burnel, P. (2017). L'impact de la T2A sur la gestion des établissements publics de santé. *Journal de gestion et d'économie médicales*, 35(2–3), 67–79.

Casey, J.T., Brinton, T.S., Gonzalez, C.M. (2009). Utilization of lean management principles in the ambulatory clinic setting. *Nature Reviews Urology*, 6(3), 146.

Cayirli, T., Veral, E., Rosen, H. (2006). Designing appointment scheduling systems for ambulatory care services. *Health Care Management Science*, 9(1), 47–58.

Compondu, C., Cheikhrouhou, N., Décosterd, I. (2018). Développement d'une démarche Lean pour la réorganisation et la planification des activités au sein d'un centre médical ambulatoire. *Actes de GISEH*, Geneva, Switzerland.

Fortineau, V., Roussel, L., Lamouri, S., Eckerlein, G., Rieutord, A., Curatolo, N., Fior, R. (2017). *Le management des flux hospitaliers basé sur les parcours patient*. CIGI, Compiègne, France.

Green, L.V., Savin, S., Murray, M. (2007). Providing timely access to care: What is the right patient panel size? *The Joint Commission Journal on Quality and Patient Safety*, 33(4), 211–218.

Gunawan, A. and Lau, H.C. (2013). Master physician scheduling problem. *Journal of the Operational Research Society*, 64(3), 410–425.

Gupta, D. (2012). Patient appointments in ambulatory care. *Handbook of Healthcare System Scheduling* [Online]. Available at: https://scholar.google.fr/citations?view_op=view_citation&hl=fr&user=DChaJ20AAAAJ&cstart=20&pagesize=80&sortby=pubdate&citation_for_view=DChaJ20AAAAJ:r0BpntZqJG4C.

Klasen, A., Fior, R., Barthier, S., Frachette, M., Rieutord, A., Barbault-Foucher, S. (2014). Le chemin clinique du patient recevant une chimiothérapie à l'hôpital de jour : en route vers le Lean management. *Journal de pharmacie clinique*, 33(2), 100–110.

Lamé, G., Jouini, O., Stal-Le Cardinal, J. (2016). Chimiothérapie ambulatoire : revue critique avec cas d'étude. *Actes de GISEH*, Casablanca, Morocco.

Pillet, M., Martin-Bonnefous, C., Bonnefous, P., Courtois, A. (2011). *Gestion de production: les fondamentaux et les bonnes pratiques*, 5th edition. Editions Eyrolles, Paris, France.

Sadki, A. (2012). Planification des chimiothérapies ambulatoires avec la prise en compte des protocoles de soins et des incertitudes. Thesis, Ecole Nationale Supérieure des Mines de Saint-Etienne, France.

Santibáñez, P., Chow, V.S., French, J., Puterman, M.L., Tyldesley, S. (2009). Reducing patient wait times and improving resource utilization at British Columbia cancer Agency's ambulatory care unit through simulation. *Health Care Management Science*, 12(4), 392.

Tohidi, M., Kazemi Zanjani, M., Contreras, I. (2019). Integrated physician and clinic scheduling in ambulatory polyclinics. *Journal of the Operational Research Society*, 70(2), 177–191.

Vahdat, V., Namin, A., Azghandi, R., Griffin, J. (2019). Improving patient timeliness of care through efficient outpatient clinic layout design using data-driven simulation and optimisation. *Health Systems*, 1–22.

Villamizar, J.R., Coelli, F.C., Pereira, W.C.A., Almeida, R.M. (2011). Discrete-event computer simulation methods in the optimisation of a physiotherapy clinic. *Physiotherapy*, 97(1), 71–77.

14

Treatment Protocols Generated by Machine Learning: Putting a Case Study of Hospitalization at Home into Perspective

14.1. Introduction

Hospitalization at home (HaH) is a form of hospitalization that allows for a range of medical and paramedical care to be performed at a patient's home. These health structures have two main objectives: to allow traditional hospitals to reposition themselves as a technical medical platform by shortening or avoiding hospitalization time, while offering the patient a guarantee of quality and continuity of care in a familiar environment. HaH also covers a range of technical and complex care, which makes it an alternative particularly suited to vulnerable populations of all ages, who suffer from heavy, progressive, chronic and/or unstable polypathologies.

This chapter examines the following issues: What are the organizational challenges of HaHs today? How can protocolization respond to them and within what limitations? How can the forecast for the trajectory and cost of the patient's stay automatically generate protocols?

Chapter written by Alice MARTIN, Jean-Baptiste GUILLAUME, Alain GUINET and Julien FONDREVELLE.

14.2. Context and perspective

14.2.1. *France's healthcare restructuring and the impact for HaH*

These health institutions were developed in France in the 1950s under the leadership of Dr. Siguier of the Ténon Hospital (Paris). The model was initially inspired by Dr. Bluestone's "Home Care" hospital in New York, created to respond to the explosion of his patient numbers (Raffy-Pihan 1997).

The model has been popular ever since, and between 2006 and 2016, 143 such structures opened in France, while the number of days spent hospitalized at home recorded per year jumped to three million (Mauro 2017). Thus, in France, HaH is continuing along its strong growth trajectory in parallel with the restructuring of the healthcare proposition. Between 2013 and 2017, 13,600 hospital beds were closed, while in HaH, reception capacities increased by 7.1%, accounting for a total of 17,400 patients who could now be treated simultaneously in the region (DGOS 2019). The 2018–2022 National Health Strategy clearly shows the desire to develop this mode of healthcare, in particular to meet the needs of an aging population who sometimes have difficulty accessing technical healthcare facilities. In 2018, HaH represented 5.5 million days spread over 213,818 stays, or an average length of stay of 25 days (DGOS 2019).

The national HaH utilization rate in 2018 was 21.3 patients treated per day per 100,000 inhabitants. In 2016, HaH represented 5% of the total number of full hospital days (Mauro 2017).

Since the circular DHOS/O no. 2004-44 of 2004, HaH has been recognized as a full-fledged hospital structure and substitute for hospitalization accommodation. Within this legislative framework, these establishments are certified by the *Haute Autorité de la Santé* (the French High Authority for Health) under the same conditions as traditional structures. HaH exists in many forms and can be public or private, lucrative or associative status, autonomous or attached to a hospital healthcare structure.

14.2.2. *Hospitalization at home and target patients*

HaH covers a total of 29 treatments. The typical patient is admitted with a primary care model and a secondary care model. This medical assessment results from the assignment of a Karnofsky Index, corresponding to the degree of dependence on care.

	Karnofsky Index
10%	The patient is dying, the fatal process is progressing rapidly
20%	The patient (very ill) requires active supportive treatment
30%	The patient is severely disabled
40%	The patient is disabled and requires special assistance and care
50%	The patient requires ongoing help and frequent medical attention
60%	The patient requires ongoing assistance and frequent medical attention
70%	The patient is able to take care of themself, but is unable to lead a normal life or able to work
80%	The patient is able to carry out normal daily activities with effort, with some symptoms or minor signs of the disease
90%	The patient is able to perform normal daily activities, with symptoms or minor signs of the disease
100%	The patient has no signs or symptoms of the disease

Table 14.1. *Karnofsky Index and corresponding health state*

In 2018, the most common form of care was complex dressing (28% of the total activity in the region), closely followed by palliative care (25%) (ATIH 2019). In addition, 1/3 of HaH days concerned cancerous pathologies. The average Karnofsky Index is 40% (FNEHAD 2018).

Principal care mode	Number of days in 2018	%
Complex dressings and specific treatments	1,573,178	28%
Palliative care	1,404,310	25%
Heavy nursing care	469,853	8%
Enteral nutrition	341,949	6%
Intravenous therapy	331,488	6%
Post-cancer chemotherapy surveillance	217,188	4%
Pain management	167,774	3%

Table 14.2. *Breakdown of the main modes of care for HaH in 2018 (in days) – source: ATIH*

14.2.3. *The positioning of hospitalization at home versus traditional medicine*

Several recent studies (Salter 2015; Leung *et al.* 2016) explore the historical positioning of HaH *vis-à-vis* hospitalized accommodation, and also *vis-à-vis* community medical practices.

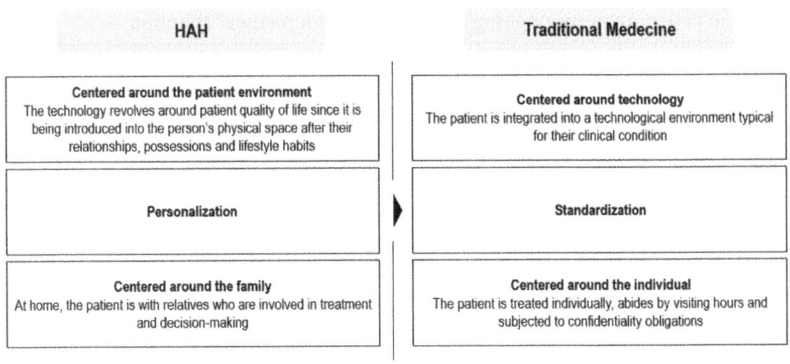

Figure 14.1. *Positioning of HaH and traditional medicine in relation to the patient and their environment*

The differences are also reflected in the costing model. HaH works on Activity Based Costing (ABC), but is also cheaper. In 2018, the average cost of an HaH day billed to health insurance was 119.7 € as compared to 184 € for conventional hospitalization. Overall, HaH will have cost the *Caisse Nationale d'Assurance Maladie* (i.e. the "National Health Insurance Fund") known by its acronym CNAM, one billion euros over the same year (FNEHAD 2018).

The interface between HaH and the rest of the healthcare network is mainly focused on the inflow/outflow of patients: admission to HaH must be prescribed by a private practitioner or a hospital doctor.

In practice, the main channel for admission into an HaH scenario is the hospital, with hospitals fielding more than 64% of requests in 2018. However, more than three out of five stays were initiated from home and prescribed by the attending physician, making it possible to avoid conventional hospitalization (FNEHAD 2018). To improve the quality and continuity of care for these patients, it is necessary to identify, on the one hand, the encouraging factors and, on the other hand, the deterring aspects, for the prescription of HaH by general practitioners.

The analytical framework proposed by Leung *et al.* (2016) suggests obstacles linked to poor knowledge of how to initiate HaH and the role of the attending physician. The article mentions in particular the time consumed by requests, information that is not directly accessible, the coordination with the HaH doctor and the remuneration for home visits. Other studies, such as that by Besombes *et al.* (2017), expose issues related to the evolution of medical practices. The shortage of general practitioners and a desire for more stable working conditions are hardly compatible with the heavy investment of multiple home visits, sometimes urgent and unscheduled, which disrupt the functioning of a practice.

14.2.4. *The problems facing hospitalization at home*

The development of HaH faces strategic, organizational and operational constraints. On the one hand, doctors prescribing admission may be afraid of engaging their responsibility for a treatment which turns out to be complex and generates significant clinical risks (Sentilhes-Monkam 2005). On the other hand, HaH experiences the same cost and efficiency pressures as conventional hospitalization. The two foremost elements for the HaH cost structure are as follows:

– healthcare services billed by private and salaried staff working at the patient's home;

– pharmaceuticals, consumables and medical devices.

Conversely, revenue comes from ABC, which amounts to a daily allowance allocated per patient according to three descriptors of their clinical condition: the primary and secondary care models associated with the Karnofsky Index. Besombes *et al.* (2017) attempt to establish a link between item costs, revenues and patient profile descriptors. The lack of correlation between these criteria shows that there are other drivers at work, for example the pathology or the social condition of the patient.

In fact, the health manager and/or coordinating doctor establishes a healthcare plan upon admission, containing in particular, the nature of the care to be provided, the frequency of visits and the nursing staff involved. In practice, many deviations are observed between the initial care plan and the care plan actually carried out. A first investigation carried out in an HaH in the Auvergne-Rhône-Alpes region suggests that these digressions may be due to the fact that the patients treated have complex and progressive pathologies that complicate the development of a reliable healthcare plan that has had to evolve since the first evaluation.

These cost and efficiency constraints require, in particular, the optimization not only of the treatments prescribed, the examinations entailed and the healthcare that follows, but also their delivery and therefore all the logistical and informational flows between the various internal and external actors. Ben Bachouch *et al.* (2012) notably remark on the issues of:

– collaboration between network actors, both during the transmission of clinical information between private and salaried nursing staff, and then again at the interface with healthcare providers such as pharmacies and laboratories;

– resource allocation and the planning of care rounds;

– information systems for the digital management of prescriptions and patient records: due to the proliferation of independent actors using the system, software training and the standardized updating of records remain two of the hardest challenges.

Independent users are also numerous since of the size of the territory to be covered requires multiple practices.

Several studies, including Chevalier *et al.* (2015), suggest protocolization as a tool for controlling costs and quality, and also as a means of improving the interface between prescribing physicians and HaH.

14.3. The contribution of protocolization

14.3.1. *A quality tool for the patient and the healthcare provider*

The impact of protocols on healthcare quality has been the subject of numerous studies in the scientific literature since their formalization in the 1970s. The protocol is defined by HaH as "the scheme of optimal care by a multi-professional medical team". Essentially, this is a set of recommendations on the best healthcare practice for a given clinical situation.

Hewitt-Taylor (2004) describes the process of writing and implementing a nursing healthcare protocol in an intensive care unit through five structured steps:

1) Establish the protocol parameters: pathologies, scope, focus group, comorbidities and potential interactions.

2) Identify a multidisciplinary development group: bringing together the disciplines concerned, numerically in proportion so as to avoid a "dominance" effect of people with a higher status being granted privileged consideration.

3) Research and synthesize the practices: possibly resulting from clinical research or patient experience, then assess their relevance.

4) Have the protocol evaluated by a group of experts.

5) Monitor protocol implementation using predefined evaluation parameters and updating the protocol regularly.

This study further suggests that protocols can benefit the expanding role of nurses by allowing them to integrate additional responsibilities as part of their skill sets.

Besombes *et al.* (2017) present the benefits of protocolization most commonly described: securing healthcare, increasing quality while making it possible to control costs, and the empowerment of nursing staff who can refocus on informal care for the patient. The protocol interface takes the form of a therapeutic handbook, stating that all the drugs typically administered in a given clinical scenario need also be determined. The support and means of communication it provides remain strong motivators for the adoption of the protocol by the nursing staff.

Other studies (Lim and Kim 2019) also express the benefits felt by the patient, in particular in situations where they are likely to undergo healthcare situations that may be stressful: decreases in anxiety and signs of depression, and overall greater satisfaction with the experience.

14.3.2. *The interface protocol between healthcare facilities*

For healthcare facilities, the challenges are not only to optimize the efficiency, quality and patients' experience of healthcare, but also to have recourse to HaH at the optimal time along the patient's journey. The role of protocol can be to relax the interfaces with the input channels, that is, private practice and conventional hospitals, by helping to clearly define the roles between the stakeholders and the patient focus group concerned.

Leung *et al.* (2016) recommend developing HaH admissions upon discharge from emergency reception services, and thus assess the patient's eligibility directly from the emergency room in order to organize their return to the home nursing scenario.

The study also recommends simplifying admission, information accessibility for general practitioners, and clarifying the roles between treatment physicians and coordination physicians of the HaH.

A study by Chevalier *et al.* (2015) reports on the implementation of an innovative protocol using laser photo vaporization of the prostate, between an inpatient department with accommodation and an HaH scenario after outpatient surgery. The nursing staff describe a reassessment and harmonization of practices, as well as better traceability in terms of the continuity of care. Healthcare providers at home can also sometimes feel isolated when looking after patients in complex situations: the protocol identifies a clinician point of contact in the event of any problems encountered.

14.3.3. *Protocol facing its limitations*

This same study discusses a number of limitations and notably mentions the existence of a link between the standardization of practices and the loss of professional autonomy. It is therefore a matter of finding a compromise between the formalization of acts of care and providing the healthcare provider the room to maneuver within their clinical decision-making capacity. These same complications are mentioned in other previous studies (Cloarec 2008). The recommendations written by a group of experts can also create a rift between "elites" and the healthcare actors on the ground.

14.4. Study and proposed methodology

Protocolization has proven itself as a tool for controlling costs and assisting in the planning of operations. We want to automate the creation of care protocols from the history of patient data taken from an HaH in the Lyon region. The study we are proposing will lead to the implementation of a bedside clinical decision support tool and will take place in three main stages:

1) identification of the cost drivers of a hospitalization at home;

2) forecast of the patient's care trajectory and costs over the course of the treatment;

3) generation of protocols for similar trajectories and the optimization of resources.

14.4.1. *Case study of the cost drivers of a hospitalization at home*

An initial analysis of the financial statements of the HaH in the Lyon region allowed us to identify the following cost structure:

– 54% of the costs are linked to direct care carried out in the patient's home, among which nursing care is the most represented.

– 20% and 9% of costs, respectively, come from the pharmacy (drugs and consumables) and the medical devices installed in the home (hospital bed, ventilator, etc.).

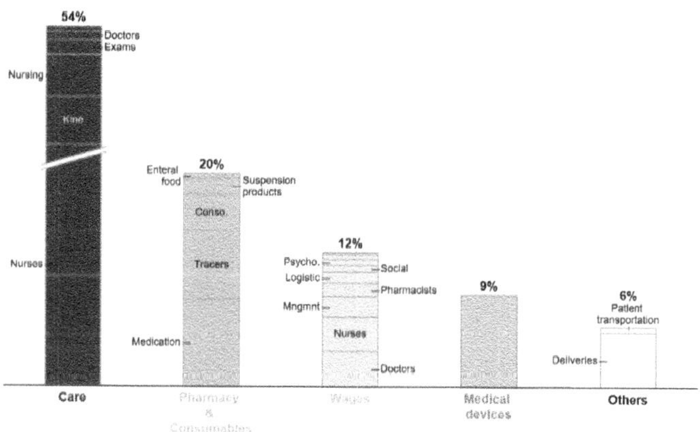

Figure 14.2. *Analysis of expenses relating to HaH "Soins et Santé" (Lyon) stays over 2018. For a color version of this figure, see www.iste.co.uk/chaabane/healthcare.zip*

This first analysis allows us to assume that protocolization could cover more than 83% of the expenses related to a hospitalization at home.

The preponderance of care activities in HaH expenditure prompted us to further quantify and analyze the costs of care in order to identify the characteristics of the patient profile that may influence this sum. The hospital partner for this study had computerized patient records for the last 20 years, from which the following information was extracted:

– Administrative data: age and sex of the patient, prescribing doctor, number and duration of stays in HaH.

– Socio-economic data: country of birth, family situation and presence of healthcare providers at home.

– Clinical data: treatment method, main diagnosis and number of associated diagnoses, Karnofsky Index and whether the patient is deceased.

Exploratory data analysis (sample of 30,000 stays) shows that the average length of stay is 50 days, and that 75% of stays last less than 52 days. The daily cost of care (the first item of expenditure) is broken down as follows: the average is 71 €/day, whereas a patient at home can generate expenses of up to 773 €/day.

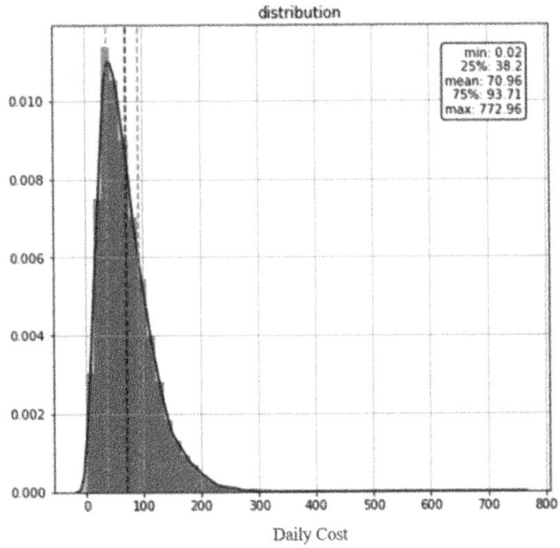

Figure 14.3. *Analysis of expenses relating to HaH stays over the year 2018. For a color version of this figure, see www.iste.co.uk/chaabane/healthcare.zip*

In fact, this variation in healthcare costs can be explained by the presence of patients with numerous co-morbidities: 73% of patients have between 3 and 12 associated diagnoses. The study of the change in the cost of the day as a function of this number suggests that this characteristic may influence the expense.

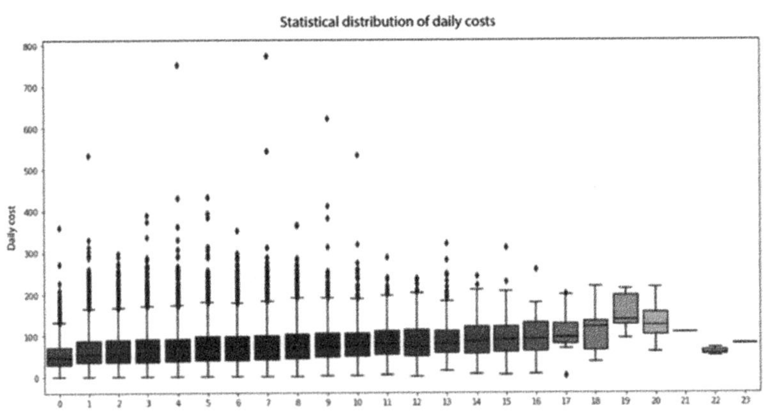

Figure 14.4. *Distribution of the daily cost of healthcare according to the number of associated diagnoses. For a color version of this figure, see www.iste.co.uk/chaabane/healthcare.zip*

To identify the characteristics of the patient profile that may also influence the daily cost, the machine learning technique of *gradient boosting* is applied (Mason *et al.* 1999). The important characteristics are the method of management with which the patient is admitted, the Karnofsky Index assigned to the patient, their age, the length of their stay, their main diagnosis and the number of associated diagnoses.

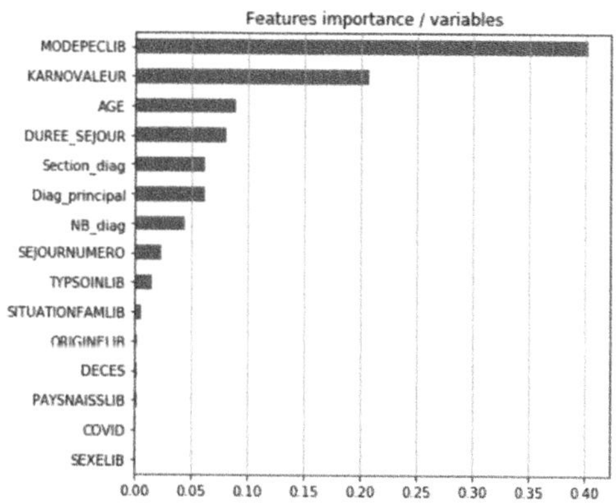

Figure 14.5. *Weighted distribution of patient characteristics in the forecasting of daily care costs*

14.4.2. *Patient trajectory forecasting and protocol generation*

The automation of clinical prescriptions has been the subject of numerous scientific studies, particularly since the development of Clinical Decision Support Systems (CDSS). We suggest studying the computational methods used for the automated generation of protocols. Why automate this process? Artificial intelligence techniques now make it possible to simultaneously take into account a large number of social–medical criteria in order to better identify patient profiles with similarities. The aim is not to take the place of the clinician, but to offer them a decision support that can alert them to specific and complex medical situations.

Machine learning is a discipline of artificial intelligence that involves extracting patterns of recurring behavior within large sets of data, then interpreting them in order to build a predictive model. The objective here is to study the history of medical data so as to extract the statistically prevalent prescriptions for the same patient profile. The following four studies each suggest a method for generating protocols and present the impacts observed if they have been measured.

Publication	Environment	Algorithm type	Impact measurement indicator
Zhang *et al.* (2014)	Pediatric hospital	Linear optimization K-clustering	Increase in the use of order sets Reduction in prescription effort
Doddi *et al.* (2001)	Public data	Association rule mining	No impact assessment
Wright and Sittig (2006)	Outpatient service	Frequent itemset mining	No impact assessment
Chen *et al.* (2016)	Military hospital	Collaborative Filter recommender	Decrease in readmission and 30-day mortality indicators

Table 14.3. *Method used and impact measured per environment in the bibliography*

We suggest developing a method in two stages as follows:

1) Group the profiles of patients treated through HaH into clinical segments showing similarities in terms of diagnoses, types of treatment, progression of the clinical condition (Karnofsky Index) and frequency of home visits by the nursing staff.

2) For a given patient, automatically affiliate their profile to a clinical segment and forecast the treatments and resources that they are likely to mobilize during their stay, which will constitute as the treatment protocol.

The second step of generating personalized treatment recommendations is fairly well-documented, but encounters two challenges in practice:

– The route that a patient is likely to take depends not only on their clinical state at time *t*, but also on their history.

– Identifying relevant recurring patterns in biased data (e.g. already existing protocol) which lack counterfactual information is difficult.

Indeed, for the algorithm to correctly identify the correspondence of a patient to a treatment, it must have both the results of the treatment on a similar patient, but also the results of no treatment. Access to groups of similar patients with different treatments can also be complex if clinical protocols are already in place.

Atan *et al.* (2018) address this problem by simulating missing data using an auto-encoding neural network. Wager and Athey (2015) reduce their data bias by using algorithmic trees that estimate, at each branch, the effect (or not) of a given treatment by assigning a propensity score. These methods show extremely promising results but have not yet been applied to real world data.

14.5. Conclusion

Hospitalization at home has experienced strong growth since the early 2000s, supported by favorable government policy and in face of the restructuring of the conventional hospital care proposition. This expansion is reflected both in terms of the number of establishments opened but also through the number of patients admitted.

However, HaH is experiencing organizational and operational constraints, particularly in terms of the management of human and material resources, cost control, and also from the new requirements of quality and traceability being placed on healthcare to which the status of the hospital is wholly subjected. The national HaH use rate is very disparate across the country and is still below the national target that has been set at 30 patients per 100,000 inhabitants. The channels of entry are sometimes poorly understood by health professionals.

In this context, protocolization seems to provide some answers to the issues raised. The benefits can be measured through numerous studies, both in terms of the impact on professional practices, but also on how the patient feels about the care received. In order to make the most of the interfaces between structures, the implementation of universal protocols is recommended. The study should make it possible to quantitatively analyze the impact of a protocol in terms of the planning of human resources and material consumption, as well as the reduction in the variability of care. Bearing in mind the economic impact, it will be necessary in particular to study the place of telemedicine, in particular teleconsultation and teleassistance within the protocol, as a prescription for healthcare in its own right.

14.6. References

Atan, O., Jordon, J., Van der Schaar, M. (2018). Deep-treat: Learning optimal personalized treatments from observational data using neural networks. *Proceedings of the AAAI Conference on Artificial Intelligence*, 32(1) [Online]. Available at: https://ojs.aaai.org/index.php/AAAI/article/view/11841.

ATIH (2019). Analyse de l'activité hospitalière 2018, champ HAD. PMSI HAD 2016-2017-2018-2019.

Ben Bachouch, R., Guinet, A., Ruiz, A. (2012). Problématiques de gestion des structures de soins à domicile : un état des investigations. *Actes Conference GISEH 2012 (6ème Conférence en gestion et ingéniérie des systèmes hospitaliers)*, Quebec.

Besombes, B., Guinet, A., Dubost, F., Marcon, E. (2017). Internalisation/externalisation de la fonction médicale. *Gestions hospitalières*, 562.

Chen, J.H., Podchyiska, T., Altman, R.B. (2016). OrderRex: Clinical order decision support and outcome predictions by data-mining electronic medical records. *Journal of the American Medical Informatics Association*, 201, 339–348.

Chevalier, L.B.J., Marquestaut, O., Lukacs, B., De Stampa, M. (2015). Impact sur les pratiques professionnelles d'un protocole de soins mis en place entre l'hospitalisation avec hébergement et l'hospitalisation à domicile. *Santé publique*, 27(2), 205.

Cloarec, P. (2008). Protocoles, référentiels de soins, démarche qualité : autonomie collective et dépendance personnelle. *Recherche en soins infirmiers*, 93(2), 28–31.

DGOS (2019). Les chiffres clefs de l'offre de soins 2018. Report, DGOS.

Doddi, S., Marathe, A., Ravi, S.S., Torney, D.C. (2001). Discovery of association rules in medical data. *Medical Informatics and the Internet in Medicine*, 26(1), 25–33.

FNEHAD (2018). Rapport d'activité 2017–2018. Report, FNEHAD.

Hewitt-Taylor, J. (2004). Clinical guidelines and care protocols. *Intensive and Critical Care Nursing*, 20(1), 45–52.

Leung, I., Casalino, E., Pateron, D., Grateau, G., Garandeau, E., De Stampa, M. (2016). Participation des médecins généralistes dans les prises en charge de leurs patients en hospitalisation à domicile. *Santé publique*, 28(4), 449–504.

Lim, H.J. and Kim, B.Y. (2019). Effects of a standardized care protocol for patients with degenerative spine disease. *The Open Nursing Journal*, 13(1).

Mason, L., Baxter, J., Bartlett, P., Frean, M. (1999). Boosting algorithms as gradient descent. In *Advances in Neural Information Processing Systems 12 (NIPS 1999)*, Solla, S., Leen, T., Müller, K. (eds). MIT Press, Cambridge, MA.

Mauro, L. (2017). Dix ans d'hospitalisation à domicile (2006–2016). *Les dossiers de la DREES n°23*, December.

Ministère de la santé, de la famille et des personnes handicapées (2004). CIRCULAIRE N°DHOS/O/2004/44 du 4 février 2004 relative à l'hospitalisation à domicile.

Raffy-Pihan, N. (1997). L'hospitalisation à domicile : une alternative également adaptée aux personnes âgées. *Actes communications au colloque SYSTED 97*, Chicago, IL.

Salter, E.K. (2015). The re-contextualization of the patient: What home health care can teach us about medical decision-making. *HEC Forum*, 27(2), 143–156.

Sentilhes-Monkam, A. (2005). Rétrospective de l'hospitalisation à domicile. *Revue française des affaires sociales*, (3), 157–182.

Wager, S. and Athey, S. (2015). Estimation and inference of heterogenous treatment effects using random forest. arXiv preprint arXiv: 1510.04342.

Wright, A. and Sittig, D.F. (2006). Automated development of order sets and corollary orders by data mining in an ambulatory computerized physician order entry system. *AMIA Annual Symposium Proceedings*, 819–823.

Zhang, Y., Padman, R., Levin, J.E. (2014). Paving the COWpath: Data-driven design of pediatric order sets. *Journal of the American Medical Informatics Association*, 21(2), 304–311.

15

Resilience of Healthcare Teams: Case Study of Two Cardiology Intensive Care Units

15.1. Introduction

Healthcare organizations are systems open to their environment, which make them particularly sensitive to external influences. They operate in an uncertain, complex and increasingly restrictive environment (Plsek and Greenhalgh 2001). To ensure better safety for patients, two approaches to risk management come together. The first, more traditional one, defines safety as a state to be achieved. Therefore, in order to manage risks and improve healthcare safety, organizations try to put anticipatory strategies into place by creating and implementing rules and protocols that are resources for action. Nevertheless, the proliferation of procedures and the standardization of practices can lead to organizational rigidity (Chuang 2013; Nyssen and Blavier 2013). The second approach corresponds to a more recent vision of safety, developed by the branch of research on organizational reliability and resilience (Weick 1993; Weick *et al.* 1999; Weick and Sutcliffe 2001, 2007; Sutcliffe and Vogus 2003). Safety is defined here as "a dynamic capability" and "an emerging property", which must be constantly reinforced given that the level of safety is never sufficient (Madni and Jackson 2009; Reiman *et al.* 2015).

Moreover, despite the various preventive and precautionary measures that can be taken, it is impossible to create procedures to anticipate all future situations and scenarios. Uncertainty is inseparable from the functioning of healthcare systems; it

---

Chapter written by Racha LAMARI.

is intrinsically linked to medical practice and can, in part, be generated by the complexity of these systems which operate in a dynamic environment (Plsek and Greenhalgh 2001). These situations challenge healthcare professionals, who must adapt and adjust to cope with hazards, while maintaining their level of performance. Resilience can prove to be an "important positive capacity" at the team level because it allows its members to improvise, adapt and bounce back in the face of significant risks (Sutcliffe and Vogus 2003; West *et al.* 2009).

In healthcare systems, and in particular within certain hospital services (emergencies, surgery, etc.), resilience is ubiquitous throughout medical practice, it is a central element of clinical work (Johnson and Lane 2016). Safety and the positive adaptation to different situations are already a part of the work of healthcare professionals. Indeed, the functioning of healthcare systems and their capacity to provide high-quality care depend essentially on their "resilience" (Fairbanks *et al.* 2014). However, this reliability can make the mechanisms through which situations are handled invisible. Attention is rarely paid to positive results. It is easier to spot the absence of resilience, by the level of system degradation and its inability to bounce back from a disturbance, than to recognize the resilience and characteristics of a resilient system (Hollnagel 2013). This is a real challenge for healthcare systems because, on the one hand it can reduce the vigilance and attentive quality of professionals and at the same time increase their feelings of invulnerability (Sutcliffe and Weick 2013). On the other hand, not all positive outcomes are about resilience. Workaround and deviance strategies can be the source of positive adaptations. A predominant use of these strategies can be counterproductive, and could result in compensating for unreliability (Wears and Vincent 2013).

In this work, we have chosen to focus our level of analysis on the healthcare teams and on the collective construction of a resilient response to changes and disturbances. Several reasons justify this choice. First, building a resilient group of people does not necessarily lead to the building of a resilient team (Home III and Orr 1998; Alliger *et al.* 2015). Indeed, social processes are crucial for the emergence of such collective phenomena. As Karl E. Weick points out, "the roots of resilience must be found in the nature of human interactions" (Vidaillet 2003a, p. 160). Moreover, despite the abundance of work devoted to individual resilience, particularly in psychology, the production of knowledge on collective resilience and on the adaptative mechanisms of teams remains insufficient. In addition, given the specific nature of the ways teams operate, the levels of analysis, both individual and organizational, do not allow us to discover the determinants of team resilience nor what makes it possible to strengthen them.

In short, detailed knowledge of the aspects relating to the production of resilient collective actions is necessary. This study aims to better understand how resilience is created, what mechanisms maintain and strengthen it, and what causes its degradation. We have chosen to conceptualize resilience at the team level as a socially constructed process.

15.2. Theoretical framework

15.2.1. *Defining the concept of resilience within the framework of the study*

The literature review on the concept of resilience reveals considerable divergences in terms of its definition, characteristics and criteria. The gradual broadening of the applied field of resilience has led to an increase in the number of bodies of works and researchers attracted by both: the multidisciplinary nature of this concept; its semantic richness and its potential application. Differences over conceptualizations of resilience are polarized around three main trends: resilience as an attribute, a process or an outcome (Egeland *et al.* 1993; Jacelon 1997; Sutcliffe and Vogus 2003; Norris and Stevens 2007; Hartmann 2016). These three conceptualizations are distinguished in terms of their theoretical implications and their methodological positions. In this work, we have chosen to envision the concept of resilience not as a "state" or "static property" of the system, but as a changing phenomenon or dynamic capacity that allows individuals and organizations to continually adjust their behaviors and responses to changes and new circumstances. Therefore, we retain the following definition: "Resilience refers to a dynamic process encompassing positive adaptation within the context of significant adversity" (Luthar *et al.* 2000, p. 543).

In recent years, research on resilience has focused more on the ability of teams to bounce back from adversity and protect themselves from the potential negative effects of stressors (Morgan *et al.* 2013; Maynard and Kennedy 2016; Bowers *et al.* 2017; Flint-Taylor and Cooper 2017; Hartmann *et al.* 2020; Stoverink *et al.* 2020). The desire to explore a level of analysis that has received little study until now directs researchers towards the need to clarify its definition, in order to distinguish it from individual and organizational resilience. Although there is no unequivocal definition of the concept, team resilience generally refers to "a dynamic [and] social process that enables a team to positively handle adverse circumstances that they collectively encounter" (Hartmann *et al.* 2020, p. 40).

15.2.2. *Nature of events and situations studied*

The starting point for all work on resilience, regardless of the discipline, is the existence of a threat. For Bergström and Dekker (2014, p. 2), "it seems impossible to define anything as resilient without something threatening its existence, functioning, or survival, at whatever level of intensity". In the literature on resilience, two major branches stand out in opposition with each other, on the question of the typology of situations that relate to resilience, or not. Some authors reserve the concept of resilience for major, exceptional, rare and devastating events (Cook and Nemeth 2006; Woods 2006; Amalberti 2013), while other researchers broaden and expand the scope of resilience to include all types of common and sometimes predictable disturbances (Braithwaite *et al.* 2017; Hollnagel and Sundstrôm 2006; Hollnagel *et al.* 2013). That is, even in situations that fall under ordinary work conditions and normal system operation, uncertainty and disturbances are constantly present and a capacity for resilience is still required (Rankin *et al.* 2014).

In our work, we have chosen to broaden our scope so as to capture all types of situations (adversity, hazards, disruptions, changes, etc.). Next, we proceed with their processing and classification according to their nature.

15.2.3. *The conceptual framework of the study*

For this study, it seems necessary for us to adopt the Weickian approach to organizational resilience because the author's thinking and conceptual tools have allowed us to approach resilience from a process perspective. Weick (Weick *et al.* 1993, 1995, 2005; Weick and Roberts 1993; Weick *et al.* 1999; Weick and Sutcliffe 2007) is less interested in organizational structures than in the processes that create these structures, in fact, organization is not the author's main research object, "rather, he is interested in the processes through which organizational reality takes shape or collapses" (Koenig 2003, p. 20). In his work on resilience, he pays particular attention to collective action and the process of constructing meaning. The author emphasizes interactions and interrelationships and favors the study of micro-processes. In addition, much of Weick's work is action-oriented. More than people, it is their behaviors which constitute the author's main unit of analysis. Weick questions the development and maintenance of a system of organized actions as a result of efforts to coordinate actions and collectively construct meaning (Allard-Poesi 2003, 2005). Under the influence of the interactionist perspective, Weick is interested in group processes, and although he devotes his analysis to interpersonal relationships, his work is not limited to the simple exchange or sharing of information, and covers at least three different levels: at the individual level, it mainly examines cognitive processes, the definition and interpretation of situations; the inter-individual level refers to the analysis of interrelated behaviors and "the dynamics of influence within them"; at the organizational and structural level, it focuses on the rules and processes that intervene in interactions, and it also takes the "systemic and dynamic nature of the organization" into consideration (Allard-Poesi 2003, p. 94; Vidaillet 2003a, p. 41). Weick is also interested in the connection between these levels, he "tirelessly tries to understand how one goes from the individual to the 'organizational'" (Vidaillet 2003b, p. 12).

In his studies on groups, Weick (1990, 1993) focuses primarily on the social processes that take place in crisis situations. He examines how in the face of extreme conditions, such as the rapid spread of a fire or an emergency aviation scenario, individuals reach a compromise on the actions to be taken, despite the different interpretations they may have on the situation.

We use the Weickian approach to resilience because the tools developed by the author seem essential to better understand resilience, both as the product of human interactions and as a dynamic process.

15.3. Research methodology

For this study, we have chosen to adopt a qualitative approach, which seems more appropriate for understanding this construct, chiefly because we consider resilience as an emerging and dynamic phenomenon (Kozlowski and Klein 2000). The qualitative study offers us the possibility of providing a more in-depth description of the phenomenon studied in a specific context, through multiple case studies (Herriott and Firestone 1983; Miles and Huberman 2003; Yin 2009), and an *in-situ* observation of situations. This allows us to investigate the relationships between context, process and outcome over time (Pettigrew 1992; Langley and Tsoukas 2016).

15.3.1. *The narrative of the event*

In this work, we are interested in near-miss situations. A near miss is defined as "a case where an accident was narrowly avoided" it can also be defined as an "error that almost occurred, but was prevented" (Le Coze *et al.* 2006). These situations allow us to better analyze the adaptability of work teams. We have also chosen to elicit and collect data through interviews, using a method based on the analysis of critical incidents. The Critical Incident Technique (CIT) was developed by Flanagan (1954) and involves "systematically collecting accounts on behavioral incidents which have been ineffective, or on the contrary, particularly effective for the success of a given activity". For this technique, it is not essential to have an in-depth knowledge of the tasks being studied (Bisseret *et al.* 1999).

15.3.2. *The data collection*

To understand the dynamics of resilience at the level of healthcare teams, we conducted two case studies in December 2019 and January 2020, in two cardiology Intensive Care Units (ICU) of two large hospitals located in Paris: *Pitié Salpêtrière* and *Bichat* (in the rest of this study, the two hospitals will be referred to by different names to preserve the anonymity of the respondents). Twenty-four semi-structured interviews with medical, paramedical and administrative staff were conducted, with each interview lasting approximately 50 minutes. We also conducted nonparticipant observations: following up patient admissions, medical staff meetings.

In this work, we have specifically chosen medical teams that provide a rich context through which to study resilience for several reasons. The working environment of these teams presents characteristics related to workload, the unpredictable nature of healthcare, the high level of interdependence between employees, and the sometimes-complex coordination of work flows (Tucker and Edmondson 2002, 2003). These characteristics meet two essential conditions for this study. On the one hand, the interdependence between members is relevant for studying a collective concept. On the other hand, these complex and dynamic working conditions offer us an ideal framework to understand how these professionals respond to different work requirements, function without errors, manage unpredictable situations and provide high-quality patient care. All of the interviews were recorded and fully transcribed.

In addition, we have chosen Cardiology ICUs because they constitute healthcare systems conducive to studying resilience, that is, they have the following two characteristics: they are both considered as secure systems in the field of healthcare safety, and at the same time, they are confronted with great variability and multiple uncertainties. We have organized our interview guide into two sets of questions covering a wide range of investigative topics: (1) team functioning (organization of work, role of team members, team spirit, hierarchical relations, communication, the conception of good team functioning according to its members), (2) the critical incident narrative (a detailed description of the origin of the event and the situation, a description of the actions of all the people who participated in the management of the event, the results of the actions taken, and the changes that were implemented after the incident). All of the information resulted in an exploitation of thematic content.

15.4. Research results

15.4.1. *Identification of stressors*

To understand resilience, we need to examine the effects of stress on team members and study how they respond to and deal with this stress. To do this, the first step of this study was devoted to identifying the sources of stress for medical personnel. From the analysis of the interviews and our empirical observations, we identified two categories of stressors: internal and external stressors.

15.4.1.1. *"Internal" stressors*

These are chronic in nature and inherent to the work of medical personnel, such as workload; fatigue, which can lead to burnout; performance stress and fear of "doing wrong"; equipment malfunction "in particular, during the care of a patient in a critical emergency" and so on. Apart from the mental burden, the physical effort is constant, especially for paramedics. In the two ICUs that we studied, the vast majority of patients are "monitored" and entirely dependent, with some suffering from a serious pathology, which makes the work of the paramedics even more difficult. In particular, this was due to insufficient staffing or an insufficient number of beds per nurse, varying anywhere from three to five, and up to 12 beds per nursing assistant:

> [...] evidently, I quit at one point because I really couldn't take it anymore [...] because we put our patients at risk if as a nurse you are caring for seven patients. It looks good on paper, but when you have two entrances to the SAMU (i.e. the Emergency Medical Assistance Service in France) happening at the same time, how do you do it? (Nurse 2, Cardiology ICU 1).

> When we are two of three at the Cardiology ICU and we have the entire Cardiology ICU full of patients to manage, it is stressful because we are afraid of doing our jobs badly... we are afraid of making mistakes (Nurse 4, Cardiology ICU 1).

> For me it's even harder [...], it really makes me crack. Physically, it's starting to get complicated (Nurse 2, Cardiology ICU 1).

> In an emergency situation like that, where the resources are lacking, or the equipment is not functioning properly, when people are not arriving fast enough, when you get the impression that the person can leave at any time, and you lack the equipment and skills around you, you find yourself confronted with these situations and you have the impression that it is slipping through your fingers (Nurse 3, Cardiology ICU 1).

15.4.1.2. *"External" stressors*

"External" stressors refer to one-off events and are related to the clinical condition of the patient. The two main factors that we have identified are emergencies and medical uncertainty. Healthcare providers in ICUs face time pressures associated with medical emergencies. Indeed, these units handle all cardiovascular emergencies, which makes it impossible to forecast patient flows.

Staff must be in a constant state of preparedness for imminent life-threatening emergencies. The second source of stress is related to medical uncertainty, which can take several forms. The situations most feared by the doctors interviewed are: (1) the difficulty of quickly establishing a correct diagnosis, given the complexity of the situation (e.g. the risk of comorbidity) and (2) the lack of therapeutic solutions when faced with a patient whose state of health continues to deteriorate.

In addition, we have observed that the operation of these units can, on a regular basis, be disrupted by spikes in activity. These temporary situations require the establishment of crisis or emergency management in order to cope with increased inflows. Most often, it results in relief measures and an acceleration of transfers between departments, depending on the severity of the patient's condition (e.g. resuscitation, or a day hospital visit). These situations also require a strong personnel mobilization, which makes delegation to junior personnel (nursing students and medical externs) inevitable.

In this study, we are interested in external threats; these events allow us to observe the relational dynamic that is put in place to manage these situations. Moreover, as Nyssen (2011, p. 235) underlines, the capacity for resilience becomes "observable and defined by the study on the dynamics of interactions and modes of coordination".

The majority of events collected did not fall outside the envelope of possible situations as imagined by medical personnel. That is, they are known scenarios within cardiology, but the time of their onset, or the form in which they occurred was unexpected. In short, the episodes were described as unforeseen and some of them highly stressful. More often than not, stressors intensify in the presence of a patient with multiple pathologies, due to the fact that the management needed for this type of patient is much more problematic. The events that have been deemed as the most stressful by medical staff are life-threatening emergencies that can have major consequences for the patient, and measured in terms of morbidity and mortality. The acute conditions or complications cited in our interviews as being the most stressful are: sudden cardiac arrest, cardiac tamponade, aortic dissection, myocardial infarction, acute arrhythmias and respiratory distress.

15.4.2. *The resilience process*

The reason for collecting the accounts of events (near-accidents) carried out using the critical incident method (Flanagan 1954) is to identify, analyze and compare the interaction processes that occur within working groups, which lead to the formation of a resilient response. Our approach attaches fundamental importance to the unique and distinct character of each individual and group response in relation to its context. This allowed us to discern comparable patterns of behavior. As a result of the analysis of our own results, as well as from our review of the literature, we have identified three phases for the implementation of resilience within healthcare teams: (1) Detection, (2) Adaptation process and (3) Results of the Collective Action.

Phase 1: Detection

Detection involves recognizing critical events, uncovering errors and threats, or simply perceiving the gap between a situation that healthcare providers expected and what they actually observed. When realized early on, detection enables faster and more effective interventions. According to Weick (2012, p. 16), the early detection of signals "increases the likelihood of recovery and continuing reliable performance". In the various accounts studied, we have noted that the signal or alert does not always manifest itself in a salient and direct manner. In addition, the process of interaction between healthcare providers and the situation may not result in the same interpretation by all group members. To illustrate these situations, at the individual and group level, we cite the following extracts:

At the level of the individual: in this first excerpt, the gap between the situation expected by the nurse and the objective situation was revealed through a conversational exchange. In other words, if the patient had not felt the pain, the nurse would not have suspected or imagined the possibility of such an error. In addition, given the atypical and improbable nature of this situation, the nurse might well have ignored the alert, or attributed the symptom to another cause. It was the patient's insistence that led her to reassess the situation. The difficult trade-off between information provided by the patient about an implausible situation and questioning the "expertise" of colleagues made it difficult for the nurse to interpret the situation. To reduce this uncertainty, she decided to collect more information needed to re-evaluate the situation. Finally, in order to avoid the possibility of repeating such a dangerous event, the nurse chose to declare the potentially avoidable event via the Osiris platform:

> [...] a patient who had an arterial catheter, while taking his blood pressure, said to me: "Oh la la! The iodine they injected in it is burning me". I said to him, "They didn't inject it, that's not possible". He replied: "Yes they did", to which I told him: "It is an arterial catheter, you puncture it, you do not inject it, it is just not allowed!" He said to me: "Even so", and indeed there was an intern, who was in his first year [...] He said to me: "Yes yes, they did in fact inject it". I said to him, "But that is a medical error". [...] I had a potentially avoidable event [Osiris] against the radiographers who had made a tremendous error by injecting iodine into the catheter [...] incompetence, an "I-don't-care" attitude, or even ignorance (Nurse 5, Cardiology ICU 1).

At the collective level: the following excerpt highlights a number of determining factors for the detection of events. First, vigilance, curiosity, and constant sensitivity to the operational context enabled the nurse, having identified the cardiac arrest, to intervene quickly. His involvement was decisive in several ways. Before his intervention, the group (the cleaner, the secretary and the nurse) were under a single construal of the event (the fall), as interpreted by the cleaner, who was on the front line when the event occurred. Using this information prevented the rest of the group from forming their own mental models of what was happening. The nurse's intervention contributed to the re-evaluation of the situation by qualified colleagues and a convergence towards a common understanding:

> [...] the cleaner saw a lady who was not very well, so much so that she fell down. So, she called the secretary who said to my colleague next to me: "Can you help me, there is a woman on the ground who has fallen". This sparked my curiosity and so I went to have a look, and in fact, she was in cardiac arrest. It's a bit annoying when people can't tell the difference between a fall and cardiac arrest. I massaged her and then I alerted other people, who then came to help us, and I said to myself: "What would have happened to that lady there [...] if I hadn't been curious?" She would have died, it is silly (Nurse 5, Cardiology ICU 1).

Phase 2: Adaptation process

In this study, we are primarily interested in the social processes that take place in particularly stressful situations (e.g. sudden cardiac arrests). We examine the mechanisms by which individuals reach a compromise on the actions to be taken, despite the different interpretations they may have of the situation. It is the emergence of organized behavior in the face of stressful, urgent and complex conditions that occupies our attention.

The following excerpt helps us to look at this question in the contrary sense, taking the collapse of the collective process of constructing meaning as a starting point (Weick 1993). In this story, the team faced a life-threatening emergency that required very rapid intervention, where the patient's life depended on it. However, no decision could have been made without the intervention of the experienced nurse. We chose this excerpt because several important ideas emerge out of this one narrative.

Faced with the inaction of this doctor who is supposed to be "*the orchestral conductor of healthcare*" (Nurse 4, Cardiology ICU 2), the nurse decided to temporarily change roles to save the patient's life, superseding the role of the doctor and his colleagues. This change of role was only possible because the nurse understood her role and that of her colleagues, and had the capacity to assume them. Colleagues who passively awaited the doctor's decision locked themselves into their official roles, which in turn restricted their freedom of action.

This situation was theorized by Weick (1993, 2003) under the term "virtual role systems". When an organization is faced with an unforeseen and unwanted event, formal roles can limit a team's ability to respond effectively (Mistry *et al.* 2015). Virtual role systems widen the individuals' field of action and allow them to free themselves from these limitations; to continue working in the absence of one or more members, and give each person the possibility of reconstituting the group in their mind, in order to play different roles (Mallak 1998). Even though the role structure breaks down and coordination is effectively shattered, members must continue to make the group function and act accordingly, given that mental simulation increases resilience (Weick 2003).

In addition, the work of the nurse and the assistant nurse has shown that the execution of complex and highly interdependent tasks relies on emerging and partially improvised coordination practices. These are informal practices that rely on interrelationships that are partly unknown and change in unpredictable ways. The way in which the situation has been handled within this team draws attention to the importance of the "emerging", "informal" and "adaptive" aspects of coordination. Furthermore, we have noted that the improvisation which is at the core of these informal practices is only really effective if it is carried out in an atmosphere of trust, or if the actors freely decide to temporarily change roles or to design and implement actions that have not been thought of before:

> [...] I was in the break room and all of a sudden three alarms started ringing. My colleague, who was in front of me, was looking, but I did not see him reacting [...] it was his patient, who was having a cardiac arrest... so I ran and... I said to him: "What is it? What we do?" [...] We were wasting time and during that time I was doing a cardiac massage ... my colleague turned on the machine and I read the VF ... a

> doctor arrived … I asked him: "What am I doing?", she replies: "I don't know". "Should the patient be resuscitated? Is there a TBR because the patient does not look well at all". […] She said to me: "no decision has been made". I said to her, "he decided for you, now you tell me and I will do it". And so, she then said to me: "I don't know" […] I didn't waste time, I told her: "We are going to apply the counter-shock". […] So I turn on the scope, but I noticed that my colleagues had made a mistake; when one counter-shocks a patient […] we have a patch connected to a cable which is connected to the defibrillator, but it was not connected, so in fact, if I had gone ahead and pressed the buttons it would have done nothing […] So it was me who had to take the cable and connect the device, charge it and apply the counter-shock […] the doctor did nothing […] And it was my nursing auxiliary, my real twin who I get along with really well, who brought me the defibrillator, and who I have now taught […] and now she knows how to do it, because she is a fast learner and is happy to learn […] I almost have more confidence in my nursing auxiliary colleague who really cares, than my other colleagues who watched me, but were waiting for the doctor's orders, when she was so paralyzed that she ended up doing nothing (Nurse 4, Cardiology ICU 1).

For comparison, we have chosen another narrative that illustrates a coordinated and synchronized handling of the situation. This excerpt highlights the collective dynamic that took place and the relational and interactive processes that have made this adaptation possible. Several factors contributed to this outcome and the successful treatment. First, the resident doctor who initially saw the life-threatening emergency remained apathetic, so as to avoid emotional contagion and avoid any spread of stress triggered by the event. The doctor tried to contain her emotions, because intense stress can be fatal to the patient, and also because it can affect the work of colleagues (as we have seen, in the preceding excerpt). Next, the interpretation and shared understanding of the situation allowed team members to anticipate the needs of their teammates (e.g. the external student went to find the head on her own initiative). This led to a quick adjustment and reduced the need for additional verbal communication. Finally, we note that the effectiveness of the team interaction process allowed for the resilient management of the situation:

> […] the patient arrived via the SAMU (i.e. the Emergency Medical Assistance Service in France), and for me it looked like a tamponade […] I […] told the paramedical team I would like to see her quickly […] so that they knew that I was in a hurry and completed their tasks efficiently, so I immediately brought the ultrasound, did the scan, and it was then that I saw that there was a huge dissection, caused by a huge adrenaline rush, I tried to stay calm so as to keep the patient

> calm to avoid a rise in blood pressure, which can cause a cardiac arrest. So I took a deep breath [...] and I asked my medical student very calmly: "Please, can you tell the nurse to bring the emergency trolley", so then she understood that it was an emergency, and so did the paramedics. Everyone understood that it was an emergency [...] so now everyone understood the situation so as not to cause a panic, and so when my boss also came he was also calm, and when he saw the file, he immediately called the anesthetist, who came immediately [...] everyone got busy very quickly [...] so the intervention went pretty smoothly [...] (Nurse 6, Cardiology ICU 2).

Phase 3: Results of the collective action

Our results reveal that, for minor events, the teams studied were able to maintain stability, no substantial changes were necessary as the consequences were minor. We noted that for relatively larger disturbances (e.g. activity spikes within ICUs), additional resources and greater absorptive capacities were required. However, after the disturbance had ended, the teams returned to normal operation. In other words, the internal operating conditions have remained stable, and the processes and structures have been preserved.

Furthermore, we were interested in the human component of these systems, which is inherently more complex and as such, cannot be conceived of as stable and constant states. Indeed, human systems are in reality dynamic "human behavior and social life are continually in flux [...] Social life is supposed to be 'in progress', never 'in equilibrium'" (Rose 1962, p. ix). This implies that these are constantly in a state of adjustment to internal and external changes (Taylor 1983; Heppner *et al.* 2004; Bandura 1997; Bandura and Locke 2003; Kofta *et al.* 1998; Tompkins and Adger 2004).

Returning to the same level of functioning means that the individual has failed to seize the opportunity and learn from the lived experience, so that the same or similar problems are less likely to recur (Richardson *et al.* 1990; Mistry *et al.* 2015). Our interviews and field observations revealed that there are many opportunities for learning in hospitals, and that healthcare teams engage in particular forms of learning. In the following, we present the different forms of learning that we have identified within the two teams.

We noted, from all of the accounts collected, that apart from the MMR (Mortality and Morbidity Review) and the various staff assemblies, meetings are infrequent. Healthcare providers communicate more through local and direct interactions:

> We share […] generally at mealtimes […] it happens as soon as we have questions, as soon as we have doubts, as soon as we have queries, we share them with the others, or if it is a somewhat complex case […] as soon as there is a striking case, as soon as there is a slightly atypical case, when there are beautiful images, a beautiful electrocardiogram, or when there is an instance of support which was particularly well executed, of which we are quite proud […] we talk about our mistakes, yes I did that, maybe I should have done that, it happens to us all (Doctor 6, Cardiology ICU 1).

> If you have a difficult charge, with a patient who is complicated, it is good to talk about it, either because it is an outlet, or because you are stressed, it helps one to talk about it (Doctor 1, Cardiology ICU 1).

These interactions and interdependencies lead to the emergence of informal practices that are essential for the collective learning process. Unplanned and unstructured discussions; spontaneous and open conversations regularly take place within the two ICUs studied. These exchanges allow group members to discuss the situations in which they are involved, share their experiences, ask questions, collect opinions, generate ideas together and explore therapeutic possibilities. The group is transformed into a receptacle for experiences, clinical case reports and sentiments. These exchanges help to develop knowledge, in order to improve current and future healthcare (see the extracts below).

We have, however, observed that these discussion spaces were limited to each professional body (medical and paramedical), and it was more difficult to engage in communication beyond hierarchical boundaries and possibly instigate a reflective appraisal of past healthcare scenarios.

The lack of inter-hierarchical meetings or discussions on these situations could have a direct consequence on the long-term performance of the team. Resilience is an important positive capacity at the team level, as it allows members to improvise and adapt in the face of potentially stressful situations in the future. Nevertheless, within these teams (in particular, Cardiology ICU 1), resilience corresponds, in certain emergency situations, to a capacity put in place *ad hoc* and are only temporary solutions (e.g. the extract – Nurse 4, Cardiology ICU 1 – cited in the "Adaptation Process" section above). The possibility of investigating or looking for the root causes, which have led, for example, to people improvising solutions in order to overcome different problems, is largely ignored. It is the same for the negative results, as illustrated in the extract below, where no effort was taken to go up the causal chain, and as such does not offer (under these conditions) any opportunity for learning. In addition, the potential of frontline actors (nurses) is not fully exploited, as they are often best placed to suggest changes to processes and activities on the basis of their relevant knowledge and the results of managing past situations, as well as their direct and permanent contact with patients, which allows them to have more balanced information.

> There was a lady who had undergone a TAVI (Transcatheter Aortic Valve Implantation), who came here […] we took her blood pressure, she is at 6 and a half […] so I say to myself: "She is not well". […] and the intern […] said to me: "Yes, give her FI 500 and then I will write the report". […] and she asks me the name of the valve, it's a CoreValve, and she asks me how it is written. I tell her: "I don't really care about the CoreValve, the lady has a blood pressure of 6 and a half". "Yes, but you give her 500 of FI and then I will come", so in the end […] I called the other intern […] the lady kept saying my leg hurts […] we told her "Yes, yes, don't worry" and so my colleague […] lifted the blanket and in fact she had limb ischemia […] we wondered if it was not from the OR that she had a white leg and if no one had seen that when they put her on the bed before bringing her to us… there was no blood circulating, so in the end we had to call the vascular surgeon […] then in the operating room […] she died […] Who missed what? I don't know […] (Nurse 4, Cardiology ICU 1).

Other types of informal discussion spaces emerged within the teams under observation. These take place when a team member experiences a strong and temporarily disabling emotional experience. This emotional impact is most often caused by the occurrence of a serious adverse event, resulting in a life-threatening situation, or even the death of the patient (see extract below). In our interviews we were able to identify that these exchanges take place in the form of dyadic discussions and aim to offer psychological support to the colleague emotionally affected by such an event. This is both a spontaneous and sporadic process that relies primarily on the existence of affinity between colleagues; the person must feel safe enough to reveal their vulnerability to a colleague without fear of negative consequences. We also noted that the respondents favored peer support to help them overcome their difficulties and continue the work, because colleagues are subject to the same contextual influences. They provide a more effective form of support as it is based on a mutual understanding of the situation. These productive discussions are doubly beneficial, because in addition to their primary purpose, they also serve as learning opportunities. Indeed, they allow the members engaged in these interactions to take a step back, reassess the decisions made and their implications, and draw from these lessons moving forward:

> […] there was this intern […] who had a case of chest pain, we all thought it was a heart attack, when in fact it turned out to be an aortic dissection, and so she ended up doing a lot of work because she did

> not make this prognosis right away. She talked to me a lot about it. I was there to reassure her [...] in the end, the patient died anyway, so it was difficult. Now every time there is chest pain, I remember, you have to think about aortic dissection [...] it's become a bit of a phobia of mine to miss an aortic dissection. At the beginning of the semester, I think about it every single time whilst following similar cases as they crop up (Doctor 6, Cardiology ICU 1).

In addition, organizational learning can be facilitated through an opportunity to confidently express oneself within the group, regardless of the existence, or not, of affinity relations. Members should be able to point out errors, ask questions or come up with new ideas without fear of possible repercussions concerning "self-image, status or career" (Kahn 1990, p. 708).

As we mentioned earlier, an essential part of learning takes place during interpersonal interactions, which makes it dependent on the quality of these relationships, and by extension the work climate. Establishing and maintaining a favorable climate is in part the responsibility of a leader who chooses to promote a sense of psychological safety (Edmondson 1999). In the interviews we conducted with clinical directors, we identified a number of behaviors necessary for fostering a sense of psychological safety, such as kindness and availability (see excerpt below). In short, depending on their management style, leadership can impact the willingness of interns and/or paramedical staff to express themselves or not:

> [...] we are not in a culture of guilt at all [...] we are the first to talk about our mistakes and showcase them, as if to say, that in medicine there are treatment risks, which unfortunately we will continue to have [...] and rather than hiding things under the rug and creating a heavy atmosphere, we lean more towards the notion of debriefing, and in any case, the intern never bears the brunt of the mistake themselves, since the intern is not responsible [...] a mistake is always a collective responsibility [...] and therefore there is no problem in talking about mistakes [...] it is never the fault of the internal it is always the fault of the senior who is with them [...] we are there to play it down a bit [...] (Doctor 2, Cardiology ICU 2).

15.5. Discussion

In this work, we aimed to identify and analyze how certain stressors can shape, and at the very least influence, a team's resilience capacity. At the end of this first step, two categories of stressors were identified: internal and external. We then compared the event accounts collected using Flanagan's Critical Incident Technique

(Flanagan 1954). These events correspond to near-misses described as particularly stressful by healthcare providers. This comparison revealed coping practices that tend to form similar patterns. This made it possible to produce a model for the team resilience process, categorized into three stages:

Patient safety depends, to a large extent, on the ability of healthcare workers to detect risks early. The effective recognition and correct interpretation of events are an essential step in the successful management of situations. This phase is decisive both for patient admissions into the unit (e.g. by internal transfer, by external transfer, from home), and for patients already hospitalized. The ability of personnel to distinguish warning signals from background noise requires a significant effort in terms of attention and constant vigilance. However, we have found that as internal stressors accumulate, their effects magnify. Indeed, the workloads, time pressures and complexity of the tasks, coupled with the requirement to function without making mistakes, the volume and the information overload, considerably increase the demand for attention, which in turn mobilizes the most important cognitive resources (Hancock and Desmond 2000). Yet neither a person's resources nor attention span are limitless. The detection phase competes with other cognitive tasks, and when resources become insufficient to maintain this attention, some nurses have told us that they opt to take sick leave rather than endanger patients.

Furthermore, successful event detection does not guarantee a correct diagnosis, as the information at hand, upon which decisions are based, may be incomplete or ambiguous. The decision-making process then becomes complex and uncertain. These stressful conditions increase the search for help within and between services (e.g. resuscitation functions as a safety net for the majority of the doctors questioned). This has the effect of increasing the frequency of communications and interactions, in order to achieve a shared interpretation of the situation, an essential step in team decision-making.

The second phase that we have identified in the resilience process highlights the role of relationship practices in building a resilient response to external stressors. In this part, we studied the different formal and informal practices that have been mobilized for the formation of resilient action. We noted that the more uncertain the situation and the greater the risk, the more the interactions intensified. The actions taken were increasingly based on emerging and partially improvised coordination practices. The analysis of the accounts collected allowed us to identify other collective coping mechanisms, such as anticipating the needs of colleagues. This process is based on a mutual understanding that allows each person to plan the actions of the other in order to better integrate their efforts within the team and better synchronize tasks. Our results also revealed that the more cohesive the group of healthcare providers involved in managing the situation, the more effective the anticipation. This situation becomes even more salient when paramedics, involved in healthcare, work more effectively when in close affinity partnerships. In addition, we have found that even beyond affinity relationships, external stressors reduce hierarchical boundaries and relational tensions that sometimes arise in the daily activity of healthcare providers. Respondents describe more cooperative operations during the management of the event.

The final phase of the resilience process revealed that there are a number of practices that continue to build team resilience after the event is over. We have identified three practices in both of the Cardiology ICUs: social support, learning, and the sense of psychological safety established by the clinical director; practices that we have detailed previously in the results section.

In this study, we realized that building resilience is possible during and after event management. During the episode, it is the effective interaction processes that play an important role with regard to a team's level of resilience, and at the end of the episode, it is the discussion spaces that provide psychological support and allow for the evaluation of actions and decisions taken and the opportunity for lesson learning. We have found that all of these practices are essential, given that attitudes, feelings and expectations from past experiences influence how people perceive, interpret and respond to environmental stimuli. In other words, the past experiences of team members are of the utmost importance; they greatly shape their future experiences.

However, we have noted that the capacity for resilience does not grow exponentially, the process of resilience is not acquired *ad vitam aeternam*, it is neither stable nor permanent. It is a "complex" and "multifactorial" process which varies, for example, according to the intensity, duration and predictability of the event. This observation agrees with the conclusion of other studies (Egeland *et al.* 1993; Cyrulnik and Duval 2006; Schoon 2006), and notably that of Flint-Taylor and Cooper (2017), who describe team resilience as having, more often than not, a transient nature, which can be influenced by changes in the team dynamic, such as the departure or arrival of a new member.

In this work, we also studied the potential consequences of stress on collective resilience. The results of this study indicate that the effects of stress are multiple and largely depend on contextual factors, individual characteristics and the structure and composition of the team. In addition, in this study we found that the overall functioning of the team is sensitive to both external stressors and the leadership's reaction to these factors (see the excerpt from Cardiology ICU 1 of Nurse 4's narrative, cited in the Adaptation Process section). First, our interview analysis revealed that physicians most often see themselves as "*conductors*", and as such, their reaction to stressful events plays an important role in teamwork. More precisely, the results of this study showed that the stress generated by the doctor could have a harmful influence on the adaptability of the team. The behavior of lower status group members (paramedics, junior doctors) is to some extent a function of the behavior and decisions of the leadership. This is one of the indirect effects of external stressors on team resilience. In addition, the physician's failure to manage stress is one of the entry points for understanding how individual factors can influence team resilience. However, part of our results offset this observation. Indeed, neither the leadership's reaction, important as it is, nor the behavior of any part of the group can predict the outcome of event management in a deterministic manner. The change of role and the successful handling of the situation by the nurse (see the above-mentioned extract), who was a part of the team involved in the management of the episode in question, demonstrate that the nurse had a resilience capacity that enabled her to resist getting bogged down and swept up in the same situation as her colleagues. The nurse demonstrated internal control and agility. The understanding of the rapid adaptation to the situation can in part be explained by her many years of experience (19 years). This wealth of experience has bestowed her with a repertoire of best-practices, taken from situations experienced over time, and upon which she makes her decisions.

In this work, we aimed to identify and analyze how certain factors can shape or at least influence a team's resilience capacity. We first studied the structuring and functioning of the team. We focused on observing the work as it is carried out, analyzing the daily tasks of the actors, in particular, the role played by the quality of interactions and relations between the members of the group on the work at hand, in turn making it possible to understand the relational dimension of resilience. We devoted the second part of this study to the analysis and comparison of event accounts, by separating the "positive" results which were "lucky" (Boin *et al.* 2010), or a factor of circumstances, from those pertaining to resilience. Our aim was to identify and describe how the individual and the group recognize, adapt and absorb variations and disturbances. Next, the behavior models that emerged from our analysis allowed us to, ultimately, describe and explain how certain decisions, actions and modes of coordination directly contribute to the formation of resilient collective action.

We conclude this discussion by presenting the limitations of our research. They are mainly methodological in nature and can be considered as avenues for future research. In our work, we chose to conduct an inter-site analysis, which aimed to transcend the constraints of particularism typical to a single-site study (Herriott and Firestone 1983). We believe that a longitudinal approach would be both desirable and necessary, as it would explore inter-individual variability and further investigate the reasons why some team members manage to effectively manage situations, while others are destabilized by these events. We recommend not restricting the examination of the causes of this heterogeneity to a study on the specificities of the different responses to a particular threat, but to instead shed light on all of the causal processes from a multidimensional and interactive perspective.

15.6. Conclusion

In healthcare systems, resilience is a phenomenon that can be observed on a daily basis. What the literature needs most is a better understanding of resilient responses to accidents and incidents that permanently threaten the work of actors at multiple levels, and how organizations can contribute rather than undermine this resilience. Therefore, the objective pursued in this work is to produce more in-depth knowledge of how a team's resilience is deployed. This study aims to better understand how resilience is created, what mechanisms maintain and strengthen it, and what causes its degradation. We have noted that collective resilience mainly relies on relational processes that are strongly influenced by the quality of interactions. Organizations must consider the major effect of this relationship, on the long-term ability of individuals and teams to absorb change and learn to cope with future events.

15.7. References

Allard-Poesi, F. (2003). Sens collectif et construction collective du sens. In *Le sens de l'action – Karl E. Weick : sociopsychologie de l'organisation*, Vidaillet, B. (ed.). Vuibert, Paris.

Allard-Poesi, F. (2005). The paradox of sensemaking in organizational analysis. *Organization*, 12(2), 169–196.

Alliger, G.M., Cerasoli, C.P., Tannenbaum, S.I., Vessey, W.B. (2015). Team resilience. *Organizational Dynamics*, 3(44), 176–184.

Amalberti, R. (2013). Resilience and safety in health care: Marriage or divorce. *Resilient Health Care*, 27–39.

Bandura, A. (1997). *Self-Efficacy: The Exercise of Control*. W.H. Freeman and Company/Times Books/Henry Holt & Co, New York.

Bandura, A., and Locke, E.A. (2003). Negative self-efficacy and goal effects revisited. *Journal of Applied Psychology*, 88, 87–99.

Bergström, J. and Dekker, S.W. (2014). Bridging the macro and the micro by considering the meso: Reflections on the fractal nature of resilience. *Ecology and Society*, 19(4), 36–42.

Bisseret, A., Sébillotte, S., Falzon, P. (1999). *Manuel pratique pour l'analyse des activités expertes*. Octares Editions, Toulouse.

Boin, A., Comfort, L.K., Demchak, C.C. (2010). The rise of resilience. *Designing Resilience: Preparing for Extreme Events*, 1–12.

Bowers, C., Kreutzer, C., Cannon-Bowers, J., Lamb, J. (2017). Team resilience as a second-order emergent state: A theoretical model and research directions. *Frontiers in Psychology*, 8, 1360.

Braithwaite, J., Wears, R.L., Hollnagel, E. (eds) (2017). *Resilient Health Care, Volume 3: Reconciling Work-as-Imagined and Work-as-Done*. CRC Press, Boca Raton, FL.

Chuang, S. (2013). Adaptation versus standardisation in patient safety. In *Resilient Health Care*, Hollnagel, E., Braithwaite, J., Wears, R.L. (eds). Ashgate Publishing Ltd, Aldershot.

Cook, R.I. and Nemeth, C. (2006). Taking things in one's stride: Cognitive features of two resilient performances. In *Resilience Engineering, : Concepts and Precepts*, Hollnagel, E., Woods, D.D., Leveson, N. (eds).. CRC Press, Boca Raton, FL.

Cyrulnik, B. and Duval, P. (2006). *Psychanalyse et résilience*. Odile Jacob, Paris.

Edmondson, A. (1999). Psychological safety and learning behavior in work teams. *Administrative Science Quarterly*, 44(2), 350–383.

Egeland, B., Carlson, E., Sroufe, L.A. (1993). Resilience as process. *Development and Psychopathology*, 5(4), 517–528.

Fairbanks, R.J., Wears, R.L., Woods, D.D., Hollnagel, E., Plsek, P., Cook, R.I. (2014). Resilience and resilience engineering in health care. *Joint Commission Journal on Quality and Patient Safety*, 40(8), 376–383.

Flanagan, J.C. (1954). The critical incident technique. *Psychological Bulletin*, 51(4), 327.

Flint-Taylor, J. and Cooper, Sir C.L. (2017). Team resilience: Shaping up for the challenges ahead. In *Managing for Resilience: A Practical Guide for Employee Wellbeing and Organizational Performance,* Crane, M.F. (ed.). Routledge, Abingdon.

Hancock, P.A. and Desmond, P.A. (2000). *Stress, Workload, and Fatigue*. CRC Press, Boca Raton, FL.

Hartmann, S. (2016). Yes, we (still) can! Team resilience at the workplace. *Academy of Management*, 2016(1), 13157.

Hartmann, S., Weiss, M., Hoegl, M. (2020). Team resilience in organizations: A conceptual and theoretical discussion of a team-level concept. *Research Handbook on Organizational Resilience,* Edward Elgar Publishing, Cheltenham.

Heppner, P.P., Witty, T.E., Dixon, W.A. (2004). Problem-solving appraisal and human adjustment. *The Counseling Psychologist*, 32(3), 344–428.

Herriott, R.E. and Firestone, W.A. (1983). Multisite qualitative policy research: Optimizing description and generalizability. *Educational Researcher*, 12(2), 14–19.

Hollnagel, E. (2013). Making health care resilient: From safety-I to safety-II. In *Resilient Health Care*, Hollnagel, E., Braithwaite, J., Wears, R.L. (eds) Ashgate Publishing Ltd, Aldershot.

Hollnagel, E. and Sundström, G. (2006). States of resilience. In *Resilience Engineering: Concepts and Precepts*, Hollnagel, E., Woods, D.D., Leveson, N. (eds). Ashgate Publishing Ltd, Aldershot.

Hollnagel, E., Braithwaite, J., Wears, R. (2013). *Resilient Health Care*. Ashgate Publishing Ltd, Farnham.

Home III, J.F. and Orr, J.E. (1998). Assessing behaviors that create resilient organizations. *Employment Relations Today*, 24(4), 29–39.

Jacelon, C.S. (1997). The trait and process of resilience. *Journal of Advanced Nursing*, 25(1), 123–129.

Johnson, A. and Lane, P. (2016). Resilience work-as-done in everyday clinical work. In *Resilient Health Care*, volume 3, Braithwaite, J., Wears, R., Hollnagel, E. (eds). CRC Press, London.

Kahn, W.A. (1990). Psychological conditions of personal engagement and disengagement at work. *Academy of Management Journal*, 33(4), 692–724.

Koenig, G. (2003). *L'organisation dans une perspective interactionniste, le sens de l'action*. Vuibert, Paris.

Kofta, M., Weary, G., Sedek, G. (eds) (1998). *Personal Control in Action: Cognitive and Motivational Mechanisms*. Springer, Boston, MA.

Kozlowski S.W.J. and Klein K.J. (2000). A multilevel approach to theory and research in organizations: Contextual, temporal, and emergent processes. In *Multilevel Theory, Research, and Methods in Organizations: Foundations, Extensions, and New Directions*, Klein, K. and Kozlowski, S. (eds). Jossey-Bass, San Francisco, CA.

Langley, A. and Tsoukas, H. (eds) (2016). *The SAGE Handbook of Process Organization Studies*. SAGE Publications Ltd, London.

Le Coze, J.C., Lim, S., Dechy, N. (2006). Gestion des presque accidents et accidents majeurs : premier bilan d'une enquête sur des sites SEVESO. *Colloque de maîtrise des risques et sûreté de fonctionnement "Risques et performances"*, Lille.

Luthar, S.S., Cicchetti, D., Becker, B. (2000). The construct of resilience: A critical evaluation and guidelines for future work. *Child Development*, 71(3), 543–562.

Madni, A.M. and Jackson, S. (2009). Towards a conceptual framework for resilience engineering. *IEEE Systems Journal*, 3(2), 181–191.

Mallak, L.A. (1998). Measuring resilience in health care provider organizations. *Health Manpower Management*, 24, 148–152.

Maynard, M.T. and Kennedy, D.M. (2016). Team adaptation and resilience: What do we know and what can be applied to long-duration isolated, confined, and extreme contexts. *National Aeronautics and Space Administration*, Houston, TX.

Miles, M.B. and Huberman, A.M. (2003). *Analyse des données qualitatives*. De Boeck Supérieur, Paris.

Mistry, S., Stoverink, A.C., Rosen, B. (2015). Team resilience: A theoretical model of teams that bounce back from adverse events. *Academy of Management Proceedings*, 2015(1), 17642, Academy of Management, Briarcliff Manor, NY.

Morgan, P.B., Fletcher, D., Sarkar, M. (2013). Defining and characterizing team resilience in elite sport. *Psychology of Sport and Exercise*, 14(4), 549–559.

Norris, F.H. and Stevens, S.P. (2007). Community resilience and the principles of mass trauma intervention. *Psychiatry: Interpersonal and Biological Processes*, 70(4), 320–328.

Nyssen, A.S. (2011). From myopic coordination to resilience in socio-technical systems. A case study in a hospital. *Resilience Engineering in Practice*, 219–235.

Nyssen, A.S. and Blavier, A. (2013). Investigating expertise, flexibility and resilience in socio-technical environments: A case study in robotic surgery. *Resilient Health Care*, 97–111.

Pettigrew, A.M. (1992). The character and significance of strategy process research. *Strategic Management Journal*, 13, 5–16.

Plsek, P.E. and Greenhalgh, T. (2001). The challenge of complexity in health care. *BMJ*, 323(7313), 625–628.

Rankin, A., Lundberg, J., Woltjer, R., Rollenhagen, C., Hollnagel, E. (2014). Resilience in everyday operations: A framework for analyzing adaptations in high-risk work. *Journal of Cognitive Engineering and Decision Making*, 8(1), 78–97.

Reiman, T., Rollenhagen, C., Pietikäinen, E., Heikkilä, J. (2015). Principles of adaptive management in complex safety–critical organizations. *Safety Science*, 71, 80–92.

Richardson, G.E., Neiger, B.L., Jensen, S., Kumpfer, K.L. (1990). The resiliency model. *Health Education*, 21(6), 33–39.

Rose, A.M. (1962). *Human Behavior and Social Processes: An Interactionist Approach*. Routledge, London.

Schoon, I. (2006). *Risk and Resilience: Adaptations in Changing Times*. Cambridge University Press, Cambridge.

Stoverink, A.C., Kirkman, B.L., Mistry, S., Rosen, B. (2020). Bouncing back together: Toward a theoretical model of work team resilience. *Academy of Management Review*, 45(2), 395–422.

Sutcliffe, K.M. and Vogus T.J. (2003). Organizing for resilience. Positive In *Organizational Scholarship: Foundations of a New Discipline*, Cameron, K.S., Dutton, J.E., Quinn, R.E. (eds). Berrett-Koehler, San Francisco, CA.

Sutcliffe, K. and Weick, K.E. (2013). Mindful organising and resilient health care. *Resilient Health Care*. Ashgate Publishing Ltd, Aldershot.

Taylor, S.E. (1983). Adjustment to threatening events: A theory of cognitive adaptation. *American Psychologist*, 38(11), 1161–1173.

Tompkins, E.L. and Adger, W.N. (2004). Does adaptive management of natural resources enhance resilience to climate change? *Ecology and Society*, 9(2), 10 [Online]. Available at: http://www.ecologyandsociety.org/vol9/iss2/art10/.

Tucker, A.L. and Edmondson, A.C. (2002). Managing routine exceptions: A model of nurse problem solving behavior. In *Advances in Health Care Management*, Volume 3, Savage, G., Blair, J., Fottler, M. (eds). Emerald Group Publishing Limited, Bingley.

Tucker, A.L. and Edmondson, A.C. (2003). Why hospitals don't learn from failures: Organizational and psychological dynamics that inhibit system change. *California Management Review*, 45(2), 55–72.

Vidaillet, B. (2003a). Exercice de sensemaking. In *Le sens de l'action – Karl Weick : sociopsychologie de l'organisation*, Vidaillet, B. (ed.). Vuibert, Paris.

Vidaillet, B. (2003b). Première partie outils et materiaux, introduction. In *Le sens de l'action – Karl Weick : sociopsychologie de l'organisation*, Vidaillet, B. (ed.). Vuibert, Paris.

Wears, R.L. and Vincent, C.A. (2013). Relying on resilience: Too much of a good thing? In *Resilient Health Care*, Hollnagel, E., Braithwaite, J., Wears, R. (eds). Ashgate Publishing Ltd, Aldershot.

Wears, R.L., Hollnagel, E., Braithwaite, J. (eds) (2015). *Resilient Health Care, Volume 2: The Resilience of Everyday Clinical Work*. Ashgate Publishing Ltd, Farnham.

Weick, K. (1990). Managing as improvisation: Lessons from the world of jazz. Lecture, Aubrey Fisher Memorial Lecture, University of Utah, October 18.

Weick, K.E. (1993). The collapse of sensemaking in organizations: The Mann Gulch disaster. *Administrative Science Quarterly*, 38(4), 628–652.

Weick, K.E. (1995). *Sensemaking in Organizations*. Sage, Thousand Oaks, CA.

Weick, K.E. (2003). L'effondrement du sens dans les organisations : l'accident de Mann Gulch. *Le sens de l'action – Karl Weick : sociopsychologie de l'organisation*, Vidaillet, B. (ed.). Vuibert, Paris.

Weick, K.E. (2009). *Making Sense of the Organization, Volume 2: The Impermanent Organization*. John Wiley & Sons, Chichester.

Weick, K.E. (2012). *Making Sense of the Organization, Volume 2: The Impermanent Organization* (E-book). John Wiley & Sons, Chichester.

Weick, K.E. and Roberts, K.H. (1993). Collective mind in organizations: Heedful interrelating on flight decks. *Administrative Science Quarterly*, 357–381.

Weick, K.E. and Sutcliffe, K.M. (2001). *Managing the Unexpected* (Vol. 9). Jossey-Bass, San Francisco, CA.

Weick, K.E. and Sutcliffe, K.M. (2007). *Managing the Unexpected: Resilient Performance in an Age of Uncertainty*. Jossey-Bass, San Francisco, CA.

Weick, K.E., Sutcliffe, K.M., Obstfeld, D. (1999). Organizing for high reliability: Processes of collective mindfulness. *Research in Organizational Behaviour*, 21, 81–123.

Weick, K.E., Sutcliffe, K.M., Obstfeld, D. (2005). Organizing and the process of sensemaking. *Organization Science*, 16(4), 409–421.

West, B.J., Patera, J.L., Carsten, M.K. (2009). Team level positivity: Investigating positive psychological capacities and team level outcomes. *Journal of Organizational Behavior: The International Journal of Industrial, Occupational and Organizational Psychology and Behavior*, 30(2), 249–267.

Woods, D.D. (2006). Essential characteristics of resilience for organizations. In *Resilience Engineering: Concepts and Precepts*, Hollnagel, E., Woods, D.D., Leveson, N. (eds). Ashgate Publishing Ltd, Aldershot.

Yin, R.K. (2009). *Case Study Research: Design and Methods*, 4th edition. SAGE Publications, CA.

Conclusion and Perspectives

Healthcare systems operate in an everchanging environment, and as such are subject to disruption and uncertainty. They must constantly face this turbulent context and at the same time must respond to an ever-increasing and varied demand. They must also anticipate patient needs and be concerned about public health. The various contributions presented in this book have shown the various opportunities offered to our hospitals, as well as our care and health establishments, in order to better face this environment and implement their healthcare missions all the while ensuring quality, a sense of security and economic stability.

The first part highlighted the optimization and simulation techniques which have been widely used by industrial organizations for many years, have appeared in hospital organizations in recent years and which provide considerable help in the search for solutions replacing manual and localized procedures. Decision support models and tools have thus been developed in order to plan an activity, simulate the impact of a decision or support managers in their tactical choices. They thus provide an objective and scientific response, making it possible to set up lasting solutions.

The second part of the book focused on the organizational opportunities offered through the integration of technology and digital technology, not only in healthcare practices (surgical robots, computer-assisted medical imaging, etc.) but also in the organization of healthcare activities. Techniques have been used to facilitate the codification of medical acts, thereby allowing for a clarification of the conditions of coverage and facilitating the work of healthcare professionals. Other contributions have proposed tools for improving working conditions by taking into account ergonomic elements or by projecting towards future environments. Robotics was not limited to replacing certain activities but rather with the view of providing additional help and support certain actions, in particular those concerning vulnerable persons.

Conclusion written by Sondès CHAABANE.

Finally, Part 3 focuses on questions relating to the management of change, thereby allowing healthcare establishments to integrate innovations in a controlled context or to anticipate fundamental questions impacting hospital life, whether for the patient or the caregiver. Supporting the shift towards ambulatory care or providing regulatory assistance opens up opportunities to better adapt to this technological context. This also makes it possible to meet the expectations of Hospital 4.0 by ensuring the appropriate conditions of care, quality and patient safety. However, we concluded this section with a central question on hospital resilience, not in terms of the resilience of individuals, but rather that of the team as a whole.

The different contributions presented, the different perspectives given at the end of each chapter, combined with the current context of the health crisis, open the door to new research opportunities. First of all is continuing to integrate technological developments within healthcare organizations towards becoming innovative organizations wherein digital technologies will have a place, not only supplying tools, but providing real assistance so as to abandon artisanal methods of planning and management. These concepts must not only be implemented within our establishments but integrated upstream in our training courses for health professionals (nursing schools, medical faculties, etc.) and also in our engineering schools and masters' programmes that specialize in industrial engineering or computing. This will allow for the establishment of a real culture of "hospital engineering", not only collaborations between the world of health and industrial engineering, but fostering true synergy. Moreover, the success of projects for the transfer of industrial methods and tools is based not only on transposition but the genuine involvement of both communities, as demonstrated by the GISEH community these last 20 years.

The second research opportunity concerns healthcare providers. We have seen that a number of contributions put staff at the center of their work when it comes to team resilience or working conditions. Human resources are the most important element in all organizations and even more so in healthcare organizations. Healthcare establishments have put the patient at the center of projects and approaches so as to ensure the quality, sense of security and continuity of care. However, without healthcare providers, administrators and healthcare professionals, these objectives will not be achieved. The health crisis that we have been experiencing since 2020 has clearly demonstrated their importance, and, as such, the resilience of our hospital systems depends on our healthcare personnel. Therefore, working on approaches that also put healthcare professionals at the center of our concerns evokes very interesting scientific issues, whether in terms of decision-support approaches, optimizations or approaches that seek to improve their work environment and conditions.

The last perspective concerns optimization, simulation and artificial intelligence techniques that can still benefit our healthcare and health service establishments, and which make it possible to use all the formal or informal information that circulates within the various services. It is particularly interesting to capitalize on the magnitude of knowledge constantly generated by healthcare practices and which can benefit other hospitals. We have seen how the whole world has tried to share their knowledge about Covid-19, and the moments of solidarity in sharing data, especially at the start of the crisis. This sharing of data and information could lead to very interesting studies with the exploration of research challenges on the resilience of our systems by applying artificial intelligence techniques that make the anticipation of healthcare requests possible, or optimization techniques to plan the allocation of the various resources as accurately as possible according to normal, strain or crisis situations, and through simulating our decision-making and seeing how this impacts our institutions.

All these challenges of research lead to strengthening the synergy between healthcare establishments, universities and research laboratories, as well as manufacturers. The hospital–university–industry trio will be able to provide answers to the perspectives identified above as well as to collaborate on scientific issues for the benefit of the entire world.

Glossary

ACA	*Consultations et actes assimilés* – Consultations and similar acts
ADC	Automated Dispensing Cabinet
AI	Artificial Intelligence
ALOS	Average Length of Stay
AMTA	*Actes médico techniques automatisés (biologie clinique)* – Automated medico-technical acts (clinical biology)
ANAP	*Agence nationale de l'appui à la performance* – National performance support agency
ATAG	Authoring Tool Accessibility Guidelines
ATC	Anatomical Therapeutic Chemical classification system
ATIH	*Agence technique de l'information sur l'hospitalisation* – Technical agency for information on hospitalization
ATMC	*Actes techniques médicaux et chirurgicaux* – Medico-surgical technical procedures
AuRA	Auvergne Rhône-Alpes
AUSUS	Acceptability, Usability, Social acceptance, User experience, Societal impact

BPM	Business Process Management
BYOD	Bring Your Own Device
CAHPS	Consumer Assessment of Healthcare Providers and Systems
CC NSS ATMC V1	*Classification commune des actes techniques médicaux et chirurgicaux* – Common classification of technical, medical and surgical procedures
CCAM	*Classification commune des actes médicaux* – Common classification of medical acts
CDSS	Clinical Decision Support System
CGA	Comprehensive Geriatric Assessment
CHN	*Centre Hospitalier de Narbonne*
CHSCT	*Comité d'hygiène, de sécurité et des conditions de travail* – Health, safety and working conditions committee
CHU	*Centre Hospitalier Universitaire*
Cnam	*Caisse nationale d'assurance maladie* – National health insurance fund
CNMM	*Commission nationale médico-mutualiste* – National medico-mutualist commission
Covid-19	Coronavirus disease
CPS	Cyber-Physical System
CSEM	*Centre suisse d'électronique et de microtechnique* – Swiss Center for Electronics and Microtechnology
DESULB	Department of Health Economics
EAWS	Ergonomic Assessment WorkSheet

ECHORD++	European Clearing House for Open Robotics Development Plus Plus
EPS	Electronic Prescription Service
ERAS	Enhanced Recovery After Surgery
GA	Genetic Algorithm
GGA	Grouping Genetic Algorithm
HaH	Hospitalization at Home
HHC	Home Health Care
HHCRSP	Home Health Care Routing and Scheduling Problem
HMI	Human–Machine Interaction
ICHI	International Classification of Health Interventions
ICSSURP	*Ingénierie conjointe de la sécurité, sûreté, utilisabilité, résilience et performance* – Joint security, safety, usability, resilience and performance engineering initiative
ICU	Intensive Care Unit
IMU	Inertial Measurement Unit
INAMI	*Institut national d'assurance maladie invalidité* – The National Institute for Health and Disability Insurance (Belgium)
ISH 4.0	Information Systems of Hospital 4.0
JCI	Joint Commission International
LNS	Large Neighborhood Search
MILP	Mixed-Integer Linear Programming
MPTP	Maximum Permissive Target Problem

MSD	MusculoSkeletal Disorders
NSS V0	Healthcare nomenclature
OMPs	Operations Management Practices
OR	Operating Room
PX	Patient eXperience
RFID	Radio Frequency IDentification
RULA	Rapid Upper Limb Assessment
S&OP	Sales and Operation Plan
SAMU	*Service d'aide médicale urgente* – Emergency medical assistance service (France)
SIR	Susceptible-Infected-Recovered
SLA	Service Level Agreement
SMEs	Small and Medium-sized Enterprises
SX	Stakeholder eXperience
SysML	Systems Modeling Language
T2A	*Tarification à l'activité* – Activity-Based Costing or ABC
TLH	Tolerance Level of Harm
TRL	Technology Readiness Level
TSP	Traveling Salesman Problem
UAAG	User Agent Accessibility Guidelines
UML	Unified Modeling Language
UX	User eXperience
VRP	Vehicle Routing Problem

VRPTW	Vehicle Routing Problem with Time Windows
VSE	Very Small Enterprise
WCAG	Web Content Accessibility Guidelines
WHO–FIC	World Health Organization – Family of International Classifications

List of Authors

Adelin ALBERT
Appui à la Recherche Clinique
et Biostatistique
CHU de Liège
Belgium

Djohra AZZI
CREGISI ESP ULB
Université Libre de Bruxelles
Belgium

Juan Pedro BANDERA
Department of Electronic Technology
University of Malaga
Spain

Sarah BARDIAUX
CREGISI ESP ULB
Université Libre de Bruxelles
Belgium

Rym BEN BACHOUCH JACQUIN
PRISME
University of Orléans
Bourges
France

Sondès CHAABANE
LAMIH UMR CNRS 8201
Université Polytechnique
Hauts-de-France
and
INSA
Valenciennes
France

Etienne COUSEIN
Pharmacy Department
Valenciennes Hospital Center
France

Quitterie DE ROLL
CRRF COS Pasteur
Troyes
France

Maria DI MASCOLO
G-SCOP
Grenoble Alpes University
France

Marie-Laure ESPINOUSE
G-SCOP
Grenoble Alpes University
France

Fernando FERNANDEZ
Computer Science Department
Carlos III University of Madrid
Spain

Julien FONDREVELLE
DISP
INSA Lyon/University of Lyon
Villeurbanne
France

Franck FONTANILI
CGI
IMT Mines Albi
France

Virginie FORTINEAU
AGEPS
APHP
Paris
France

Véronique GONCETTE
Pharmacie hospitalière
CHU de Liège
Belgium

Wilson GOUDALO
ABERDI Inc.
Westmount
Canada

Didier GOURC
CGI
IMT Mines Albi
Toulouse University
France

Yohan GUERRIER
LAMIH UMR CNRS 8201
Université Polytechnique
Hauts-de-France
Valenciennes
France

Jean-Baptiste GUILLAUME
IAC Partners
Paris
France

Alain GUINET
DISP
INSA Lyon/University of Lyon
Villeurbanne
France

Khalid HACHEMI
Université d'Oran 2
Mohamed Ben Ahmed
Oran
Algeria

Antoine HAYEK
ProcSim
Lausanne
Switzerland

Djilali IDOUGHI
Université Abderrahmane
Mira de Béjaïa
Algeria

Ana IGLESIAS
Computer Science Department
Carlos III University of Madrid
Spain

Michel JEANNEY
Centre Hospitalier de Narbonne
France

Philippe KOLH
Gestion du Système d'Information
CHU de Liège
Belgium

Christophe KOLSKI
LAMIH UMR CNRS 8201
Université Polytechnique
Hauts-de-France
Valenciennes
France

Racha LAMARI
CEROS
Paris Nanterre University
France

Karine LAN HING TING
UR LIST3N/M2S
University of Technology of Troyes
France

Yoann LEBRUN
CCI Grand Hainaut
Valenciennes
France

Pol LECLERCQ
GEDIS & CREGISI ESP ULB
Université Libre de Bruxelles
Belgium

Sophie LEPREUX
LAMIH UMR CNRS 8201
Université Polytechnique
Hauts-de-France
Valenciennes
France

Nathalie MAES
Appui à la Recherche Clinique
et Biostatistique
CHU de Liège
Belgium

Didier MAESEN
Pharmacie hospitalière
CHU de Liège
Belgium

Rebeca MARFIL
Department of Electronic Technology
University of Malaga
Spain

François MARMIER
ICube UMR-CNRS 7357
BETA UMR-CNRS 7522
University of Strasbourg
France

Alice MARTIN
DISP
INSA Lyon/University of Lyon
Villeurbanne
France

Cléa MARTINEZ
CGI
IMT Mines Albi
France

Denis MENAGER
CHU de Liège
Belgium

Magali PIRSON
CREGISI ESP ULB
Université Libre de Bruxelles
Belgium

Jérôme RADUREAU
Adomni–Quemera
Bourgoin-Jallieu
France

Leah RIFI
CGI
IMT Mines ALbi
France

Valentin ROCHAT
ProcSim
Lausanne
Switzerland

Lucie ROUSSEL
APHP
Paris
France

Laurence SEIDEL
Appui à la Recherche Clinique et Biostatistique
CHU de Liège
Belgium

Sophie STREEL
Pharmacie hospitalière
CHU de Liège
Belgium

Karim TOULOUM
Université Abderrahmane Mira de Béjaïa
Algeria

Jihene TOUNSI
SMART Laboratory
Tunis University
Sousse
Tunisia

Julie VAN DEN BULCKE
CREGISI ESP ULB
Université Libre de Bruxelles
Belgium

Frédéric VANDERHAEGEN
LAMIH UMR CNRS 8201
Université Polytechnique Hauts-de-France
Valenciennes
France

Nicolas VISPI
ARACT Hauts-de-France
Lille
France

Dimitri VOILMY
UR LIST3N/M2S
University of Technology of Troyes
France

Philippe WIESER
EPFL
Switzerland
and
École des Ponts ParisTech
France

Index

P, Q, R

S, T, U, W

Other titles from

iSTE

in

Health Engineering and Society

2021

BÉRANGER Jérôme
Societal Responsibility of Artificial Intelligence: Towards an Ethical and Eco-responsible AI
(Technological Prospects and Social Applications Set – Volume 4)

CORDELIER Benoit, GALIBERT Olivier
Digital Health Communications
(Technological Prospects and Social Applications Set – Volume 5)

NADOT Michel
Discipline of Nursing: Three-time Knowledge

2020

BARBET Jacques, FOUCQUIER Adrien, THOMAS Yves
Therapeutic Progress in Oncology: Towards a Revolution in Cancer Therapy?
(Health and Patients Set – Volume 2)

MORILLON Laurent, CLAVIER Viviane
Health Research Practices in a Digital Context
(Health Information Set – Volume 4)

PAILLIART Isabelle
New Territories in Health
(Health Information Set – Volume 3)

2019

CLAVIER Viviane, DE OLIVEIRA Jean-Philippe
Food and Health: Actor Strategies in Information and Communication
(Health Information Set – Volume 2)

PIZON Frank
Health Education and Prevention
(Health and Patients Set – Volume 1)

2018

HUARD Pierre
The Management of Chronic Diseases: Organizational Innovation and Efficiency

PAGANELLI Céline
Confidence and Legitimacy in Health Information and Communication
(Health Information Set – Volume 1)

2017

PICARD Robert
Co-design in Living Labs for Healthcare and Independent Living: Concepts, Methods and Tools

2015

BÉRANGER Jérôme
Medical Information Systems Ethics

Printed and bound by CPI Group (UK) Ltd, Croydon, CR0 4YY

13/09/2026

14961037-0006